Y0-BRV-525

Food Safety
SOURCEBOOK

Health Reference Series

First Edition

Food Safety
SOURCEBOOK

Basic Consumer Health Information about the Safe Handling of Meat, Poultry, Seafood, Eggs, Fruit Juices, and Other Food Items, and Facts about Pesticides, Drinking Water, Food Safety Overseas, and the Onset, Duration, and Symptoms of Foodborne Illnesses, Including Types of Pathogenic Bacteria, Parasitic Protozoa, Worms, Viruses, and Natural Toxins; Along with the Role of the Consumer, the Food Handler, and the Government in Food Safety; a Glossary, and Resources for Additional Help and Information

Edited by
Dawn D. Matthews

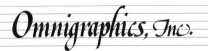

Penobscot Building / Detroit, MI 48226

Bibliographic Note

Because this page cannot legibly accommodate all the copyright notices, the Bibliographic Note portion of the Preface constitutes an extension of the copyright notice.

Beginning with books published in 1999, each new volume of the *Health Reference Series* will be individually titled and called a "First Edition." Subsequent updates will carry sequential edition numbers. To help avoid confusion and to provide maximum flexibility in our ability to respond to informational needs, the practice of consecutively numbering each volume will be discontinued.

Edited by Dawn D. Matthews

Health Reference Series

Karen Bellenir, *Series Editor*
Peter D. Dresser, *Managing Editor*
Joan Margeson, *Research Associate*
Dawn Matthews, *Verification Assistant*
Margaret Mary Missar, *Research Coordinator*
Jenifer Swanson, *Research Associate*

Omnigraphics, Inc.

Matthew P. Barbour, *Vice President, Operations*
Laurie Lanzen Harris, *Vice President, Editorial Director*
Kevin Hayes, *Production Coordinator*
Thomas J. Murphy, *Vice President, Finance and Comptroller*
Peter E. Ruffner, *Senior Vice President*
Jane J. Steele, *Marketing Consultant*

Frederick G. Ruffner, Jr., Publisher

Library of Congress Cataloging-in-Publication Data

Food safety sourcebook ; basic consumer health information about the
    safe handling of meat . . . / edited by Dawn D. Matthews. — 1st ed.
      p. cm. — (Health reference series)
    Includes bibliographical references.
    ISBN 0-7808-0326-4 (lib. bdg. ; alk. paper)
      1. Food adulteration and inspection. 2. Food industry and trade —
Safety measures. I. Matthews, Dawn. II. Series ; Health reference
series (Unnumbered)
TX531.F5685 1999   99-37611
363. 19'2—dc21   CIP

∞

This book is printed on acid-free paper meeting the ANSI Z39.48 Standard. The infinity symbol that appears above indicates that the paper in this book meets that standard.

Printed in the United States

Table of Contents

Preface ix

Part I: Introduction to Food Safety

Chapter 1 — Emerging Foodborne Diseases:
               An Evolving Public Health Challenge 3
Chapter 2 — A Guide to Safe Food Handling 23
Chapter 3 — The Color of Meat and Poultry 33
Chapter 4 — Critical Steps toward Safer Seafood 39
Chapter 5 — Safer Eggs: Laying the Groundwork 47
Chapter 6 — Critical Controls for Juice Safety 55
Chapter 7 — Pesticides in Foods 61
Chapter 8 — Should "Pre-Washed" Salad Greens Be
               Washed Again? 67
Chapter 9 — Possible Danger in Public Drinking Water 71
Chapter 10 — Don't Get Bitten by the Travel Bug:
               Eat Safely Overseas 75

Part II: Common Foodborne Pathogens

Chapter 11 — Onset, Duration, and Symptoms of
               Foodborne Illness 81

Pathogenic Bacteria

Chapter 12 — *Salmonella* 89

Chapter 13—*Campylobacter* 95
Chapter 14—*Listeria* 99
Chapter 15—*Bacillus* 103
Chapter 16—*Plesiomonas Shigelloides* 109
Chapter 17—*Shigella* 113
Chapter 18—*Streptococcus* 117
Chapter 19—Enterotoxigenic *Escherichia Coli* 121
Chapter 20—Enteropathogenic *Escherichia Coli* 125
Chapter 21—*Escherichia Coli* 0157:H7 129
Chapter 22—Enteroinvasive *Escherichia Coli* 135

Parasitic Protozoa and Worms

Chapter 23—*Giardia Lamblia* 139
Chapter 24—*Cryptosporidium* 143
Chapter 25—*Anisakis Simplex* and Related Worms 147
Chapter 26—*Acanthamoeba, Naegleria Fowleri* and
            Other Amobae 151

Viruses

Chapter 27—Hepatitis A Virus 155
Chapter 28—Rotavirus 159

Natural Toxins

Chapter 29—Various Shellfish-Associated Toxins 163
Chapter 30—Scombrotoxin 167
Chapter 31—Tetrodotoxin 171
Chapter 32—Mushroom Toxins 175
Chapter 33—Phytohaemagglutinin 187
Chapter 34—Grayanotoxin 191

Part III: The Consumer's Role in Food Safety

Chapter 35—Home-Based Food-Borne Illness 197
Chapter 36—Can Your Kitchen Pass the Food Safety
            Test? 201
Chapter 37—Sponges, Sinks, and Rags 209
Chapter 38—Slow Cooker Safety 215
Chapter 39—Freezing 219

Chapter 40—Safe Food to Go 227
Chapter 41—Advice for Packing Safe School Lunches 231
Chapter 42—Keep Your Baby Safe 233

Part IV: The Food Handler's Role in Food Safety

Chapter 43—A Menu of Modern Safety Standards 237
Chapter 44—The Impact of Consumer Demands and
           Trends on Food Processing 243
Chapter 45—Food Product Dating 247
Chapter 46—Foodborne Illnesses in the Child Care
           Setting 253
Chapter 47—In Day-Care Centers, Cleanliness Is a Must 257

Part V: The Government's Role in Food Safety

Chapter 48—Progress Report for Food and Drug Safety 265
Chapter 49—Foodborne Diseases Active Surveillance
           Network (FoodNet) 269
Chapter 50—National Computer Network in Place to
           Combat Foodborne Illness (PulseNet) 273

Part VI: Additional Help and Resources

Chapter 51—Glossary 279
Chapter 52—Food Safety: A Team Approach 293
Chapter 53—What to Do If You Have a Problem with
           Food Products 303
Chapter 54—Obtaining the 1999 Food Code 307

Index **311**

Preface

About This Book

The food supply in the United States is among the safest in the world, but foodborne infections still cause millions of illnesses every year according to government estimates. Although many people associate food-related diseases with diarrhea and vomiting, the effects can be much more serious, including miscarriage, reactive arthritis, acute paralysis, and syndromes leading to kidney failure. In addition, as many as 9,000 Americans, primarily the elderly, the ill, and the very young, die annually as a result of such diseases as *E. coli, Salmonella, Cryptosporidium,* and Hepatitis A. Consumer education about basic food safety principles is an important component of prevention.

The *Food Safety Sourcebook* describes the onset, symptoms, and duration of the most commonly encountered types of foodborne bacteria, parasites, worms, viruses, and natural toxins. It offers tips to the consumer about safe food-handling practices and provides information about government guidelines and programs to insure food safety. A glossary and other resources for additional help and information are also provided.

How to Use This Book

This book is divided into parts and chapters. Parts focus on broad areas of interest. Chapters are devoted to single topics within a part.

Part I: Introduction to Food Safety describes some common ways that foodborne illnesses are encountered and offers basic information about these dangers.

Part II: Common Foodborne Pathogens gives information on many of the common bacteria, viruses, natural toxins, protozoa and worms that cause food-related illness.

Part III: The Consumer's Role in Food Safety features chapters designed to help the consumer maintain food safety, including information about sponges and sink rags, slow cooker safety, frozen food safety, and packing school lunches. A quiz will enable readers to check the food safety standards of their own kitchens.

Part IV: The Food Handler's Role in Food Safety includes information on the standards that must be met by food handlers and food processors, along with standards for child care and day care centers.

Part V: The Government's Role in Food Safety describing the agencies that are in place to track and combat foodborne illnesses, including FoodNet and PulseNet.

Part VI: Additional Help and Resources includes a glossary of important terms, information on what to do if you have a problem with food products, a list of government agencies that work together to provide information on food safety, and information on how to obtain the U.S. Food and Drug Administration Food Code.

Bibliographic Note

This volume contains documents and excerpts from publications issued by the following government agencies: U.S. Department of Agriculture (USDA); U.S. Food and Drug Administration (FDA); U.S. Department of Health and Human Services (DHHS); Centers for Disease Control and Prevention (CDC); Food Safety and Inspection Service (FSIS); and the National Institute of Diabetes and Digestive and Kidney Diseases (NIDDK).

In addition, this volume contains copyrighted articles from *Environmental Nutrition, InteliHealth* (Johns Hopkins University), *Science News, Prepared Foods,* and *The Tufts University Health & Nutrition Letter.*

Full citation information is provided on the first page of each chapter. Every effort has been made to secure all necessary rights to reprint the copyrighted material. If any omissions have been made, please contact Omnigraphics to make corrections for future editions.

Acknowledgements

Many thanks to Peter Dresser and Omnigraphics for this exciting opportunity, to Karen Bellenir for her infinite patience and guidance in this process, and to Mark, Rachel and Jodi for their encouragement as I approached this "fork in the road."

Note from the Editor

This book is part of Omnigraphics' *Health Reference Series*. The series provides basic information about a broad range of medical concerns. It is not intended to serve as a tool for diagnosing illness, in prescribing treatments, or as a substitute for the physician/patient relationship. All persons concerned about medical symptoms or the possibility of disease are encouraged to seek professional care from an appropriate health care provider.

Our Advisory Board

The *Health Reference Series* is reviewed by an Advisory Board comprised of librarians from public, academic, and medical libraries. We would like to thank the following board members for providing guidance to the development of this series:

Nancy Bulgarelli, William Beaumont Hospital Library, Royal Oak, MI

Karen Imarasio, Bloomfield Township Public Library, Bloomfield Township, MI

Karen Morgan, Mardigian Library, University of Michigan, Dearborn, MI

Rosemary Orlando, St. Clair Shores Public Library, St. Clair Shores, MI

Health Reference Series *Update Policy*

The inaugural book in the *Health Reference Series* was the first edition of *Cancer Sourcebook* published in 1992. Since then, the *Series* has been enthusiastically received by librarians and in the medical community. In order to maintain the standard of providing high-quality health information for the lay person, the editorial staff at Omnigraphics felt it was necessary to implement a policy of updating volumes when warranted.

Medical researchers have been making tremendous strides, and the challenge to stay current with the most recent advances is one our editors take seriously. Each decision to update a volume will be made on an individual basis. Some of the considerations will include how much new information is available and the feedback we receive from people who use the books. If there's a topic you would like to see added to the update list, or an area of medical concern you feel has not been adequately addressed, please write to:

Editor
Health Reference Series
Omnigraphics, Inc.
2500 Penobscot Bldg.
Detroit, MI 48226

The commitment to providing on-going coverage of important medical developments has also led to some technical changes in the *Health Reference Series*. Beginning with books published in 1999, each new volume will be individually titled and called a "First Edition." Subsequent updates will carry sequential edition numbers. To help avoid confusion and to provide maximum flexibility in our ability to respond to informational needs, the practice of consecutively numbering each volume will be discontinued.

Part One

Introduction to Food Safety

Chapter 1

Emerging Foodborne Diseases: An Evolving Public Health Challenge

The epidemiology of foodborne disease is changing. New pathogens have emerged, and some have spread worldwide. Many, including *Salmonella, Escherichia coli* O157:H7, *Campylobacter*, and *Yersinia enterocolitica*, have reservoirs in healthy food animals, from which they spread to an increasing variety of foods. These pathogens cause millions of cases of sporadic illness and chronic complications, as well as large and challenging outbreaks over many states and nations. Improved surveillance that combines rapid subtyping methods, cluster identification, and collaborative epidemiologic investigation can identify and halt large, dispersed outbreaks. Outbreak investigations and case-control studies of sporadic cases can identify sources of infection and guide the development of specific prevention strategies. Better understanding of how pathogens persist in animal reservoirs is also critical to successful long-term prevention. In the past, the central challenge of foodborne disease lay in preventing the contamination of human food with sewage or animal manure. In the future, prevention of foodborne disease will increasingly depend on controlling contamination of feed and water consumed by the animals themselves.

Every year, in the United States foodborne infections cause millions of illnesses and thousands of deaths; most infections go undiagnosed and unreported. As the epidemiology of foodborne infections evolves, old scenarios and solutions need to be updated. This chapter

Emerging Infectious Diseases, Vol. 3 No. 4, October-December 1997, updated December 1998, Centers for Disease Control and Prevention, Atlanta, Georgia, USA.

reviews main trends in the evolution of foodborne disease epidemiology and their effect on surveillance and prevention activities.

Preventing foodborne disease is a multifaceted process, without simple and universal solutions. For most foodborne pathogens, no vaccines are available. Consumer education about basic principles of food safety, an important component of prevention, by itself is insufficient. Food reaches the consumer through long chains of industrial production, in which many opportunities for contamination exist. The general strategy of prevention is to understand the mechanisms by which contamination and disease transmission can occur well enough to interrupt them. An outbreak investigation or epidemiologic study should go beyond identifying a suspected food and pulling it from the shelf to defining the chain of events that allowed contamination with an organism in large enough numbers to cause illness. We learn from the investigation what went wrong, in order to devise strategies to prevent similar events in the future. Although outbreaks make the news, most foodborne infections occur as individual or sporadic cases. Therefore, the sources of sporadic cases must also be investigated and understood.

Emerging Foodborne Pathogens

Substantial progress has been made in preventing foodborne diseases. For example, typhoid fever, extremely common at the beginning of the 20th century, is now almost forgotten in the United States. It was conquered in the preantibiotic era by disinfection of drinking water, sewage treatment, milk sanitation and pasteurization, and shellfish bed sanitation. Similarly, cholera, bovine tuberculosis, and trichinosis have also been controlled in the United States. However, new foodborne pathogens have emerged. Among the first of these were infections caused by nontyphoid strains of Salmonella, which have increased decade by decade since World War II. In the last 20 years, other infectious agents have been either newly described or newly associated with foodborne transmission.

- *Campylobacter jejuni*
- *Campylobacter fetus ssp. fetus*
- *Cryptosporidium parvum*
- *Cyclospora cayetanensis*
- *Escherichia coli* O157:H7 and related *E. coli* (e.g., O111:NM, O104:H21)
- *Listeria monocytogenes*

- Norwalk-like viruses
- *Nitzschia pungens* (cause of amnesic shellfish poisoning)
- *Salmonella Enteritidis*
- *Salmonella Typhimurium* DT 104
- *Vibro cholerae* 01
- *Vibrio vulnificus*
- *Vibrio parahaemolyticus*
- *Yersinia enterocolitica*

Vibrio vulnificus, Escherichia coli O157:H7, and *Cyclospora cayetanensis* are examples of newly described pathogens that often are foodborne. *V. vulnificus* was identified in the bloodstream of persons with underlying liver disease who had fulminant infections after eating raw oysters or being exposed to seawater; this organism lives in the sea and can be a natural summertime commensal organism in shellfish.[1] *E. coli* O157:H7 was first identified as a pathogen in 1982 in an outbreak of bloody diarrhea traced to hamburgers from a fast-food chain[2]; it was subsequently shown to have a reservoir in healthy cattle[3]. *Cyclospora*, known previously as a cyanobacterialike organism, received its current taxonomic designation in 1992 and emerged as a foodborne pathogen in outbreaks traced to imported Guatemalan raspberries in 1996[4,5]. The similarity of *Cyclospora* to *Eimeria* coccidian pathogens of birds suggests an avian reservoir[4,5].

Some known pathogens have only recently been shown to be predominantly foodborne. For example, *Listeria monocytogenes* was long known as a cause of meningitis and other invasive infections in immunocompromised hosts. How these hosts became infected remained unknown until a series of investigations identified food as the most common source[6]. Similarly, *Campylobacter jejuni* was known as a rare opportunistic bloodstream infection until veterinary diagnostic methods used on specimens from humans showed it was a common cause of diarrheal illness[7]. Subsequent epidemiologic investigations implicated poultry and raw milk as the most common sources of sporadic cases and outbreaks, respectively[8]. *Yersinia enterocolitica*, rare in the United States but a common cause of diarrheal illness and pseudoappendicitis in northern Europe and elsewhere, is now known to be most frequently associated with undercooked pork[9].

These foodborne pathogens share a number of characteristics. Virtually all have an animal reservoir from which they spread to humans; that is, they are foodborne zoonoses. In marked contrast to many established zoonoses, these new zoonoses do not often cause illness in the infected host animal. The chicken with lifelong ovarian infection with *Salmonella* serotype Enteritidis, the calf carrying *E. coli* O157:H7, and the oyster carrying Norwalk virus or *V. vulnificus* appear healthy; therefore, public health concerns must now include apparently healthy animals. Limited existing research on how animals acquire and transmit emerging pathogens among themselves often implicates contaminated fodder and water; therefore, public health concerns must now include the safety of what food animals themselves eat and drink.

For reasons that remain unclear, these pathogens can rapidly spread globally. For example, *Y. enterocolitica* spread globally among pigs in the 1970s[10]; *Salmonella* serotype Enteritidis appeared simultaneously around the world in the 1980s[11]; and *Salmonella* Typhimurium Definitive Type (DT) 104 is now appearing in North America, Europe, and perhaps elsewhere[12]; therefore, public health concerns must now include events happening around the world, as harbingers of what may appear here.

Many emerging zoonotic pathogens are becoming increasingly resistant to antimicrobial agents, largely because of the widespread use of antibiotics in the animal reservoir. For example, *Campylobacter* isolated from human patients in Europe is now increasingly resistant to fluoroquinolones, after these agents were introduced for use in animals[13]. Salmonellae have become increasing resistant to a variety of antimicrobial agents in the United States[14]; therefore, public health concerns must include the patterns of antimicrobial use in agriculture as well as in human medicine.

The foods contaminated with emerging pathogens usually look, smell, and taste normal, and the pathogen often survives traditional preparation techniques: *E. coli* O157:H7 in meat can survive the gentle heating that a rare hamburger gets[15]; *Salmonella* Enteritidis in eggs survives in an omelette[16]; and Norwalk virus in oysters survives gentle steaming[17]. Following standard and traditional recipes can cause illness and outbreaks. Contamination with the new foodborne zoonoses eludes traditional food inspection, which relies on visual identification of foodborne hazards. These pathogens demand new control strategies, which would minimize the likelihood of contamination in the first place. The rate at which new pathogens have been identified suggests that many more remain to be discovered. Many of the foodborne infections of the future are likely to arise from the animal reservoirs from which we draw our food supply.

Once a new foodborne disease is identified, a number of critical questions need to be answered to develop a rational approach to prevention: What is the nature of the disease? What is the nature of the pathogen? What are simple ways to easily identify the pathogen and diagnose the disease? What is the incidence of the infection? How can the disease be treated? Which foods transmit the infection? How does the pathogen get into the food, and how well does it persist there? Is there is an animal reservoir? How do the animals themselves become infected? How can the disease be prevented? Does the prevention strategy work?

The answers to these questions do not come rapidly. Knowledge accumulates gradually, as a result of detailed scientific investigations, often conducted during outbreaks[18]. After 15 years of research, we know a great deal about infections with *E. coli* O157:H7, but we still do not know how best to treat the infection, nor how the cattle (the principal source of infection for humans) themselves become infected. Better slaughter procedures and pasteurization of milk are useful control strategies for this pathogen in meat and milk, as irradiation of meat may be in the future. More needs to be learned: for example, it remains unclear how best to prevent this organism from contaminating lettuce or apple juice. For more recently identified agents, even less is known.

New Food Vehicles of Transmission

Along with new pathogens, an array of new food vehicles of transmission have been implicated in recent years. Traditionally, the food implicated in a foodborne outbreak was undercooked meat, poultry or seafood, or unpasteurized milk. Now, additional foods previously thought safe are considered hazardous. For example, for centuries, the internal contents of an egg were presumed safe to eat raw. However, epidemic *Salmonella* Enteritidis infection among egg-laying flocks indicates that intact eggs may have internal contamination with this *Salmonella* serotype. Many outbreaks are caused by contaminated shell eggs, including eggs used in such traditional recipes as eggnog and Caesar salad, lightly cooked eggs in omelets and French toast, and even foods one would presume thoroughly cooked, such as lasagna and meringue pie[19,20]. *E. coli* O157:H7 has caused illness through an ever-broadening spectrum of foods, beyond the beef and raw milk that are directly related to the bovine reservoir. In 1992, an outbreak caused by apple cider showed that this organism could be transmitted through a food with a pH level of less than 4.0, possibly after contact of fresh produce with manure[21]. A recent outbreak traced to venison jerky suggests a wild deer reservoir, so both cattle and feral deer manure are of concern[22]. Imported raspberries contaminated with *Cyclospora* caused an epidemic in the United States in 1996, possibly because contaminated surface water was used to spray the berries with fungicide before harvest[5]. Norwalklike viruses, which appear to have a human reservoir, have contaminated oysters harvested from pristine waters by oyster catchers who did not use toilets with holding tanks on their boats and were themselves the likely source of the virus[23].

The new food vehicles of disease share several features. Contamination typically occurs early in the production process, rather than just before consumption. Because of consumer demand and the global food market, ingredients from many countries may be combined in a single dish, which makes the specific source of contamination difficult to trace. These foods have fewer barriers to microbial growth, such as salt, sugar, or preservatives; therefore, simple transgressions can make the food unsafe. Because the food has a short shelf life, it may often be gone by the time the outbreak is recognized; therefore, efforts to prevent contamination at the source are very important.

An increasing, though still limited, proportion of reported foodborne outbreaks are being traced to fresh produce[24]. A series of outbreaks recently investigated by the Centers for Disease Control and Prevention (CDC) has linked a variety of pathogens to fresh fruits and vegetables harvested in the United States and elsewhere (Table 1.1). The investigations have often been triggered by detection of more cases than expected of a rare serotype of *Salmonella* or *Shigella* or by diagnosis of a rare infection like cyclosporiasis. Outbreaks caused by common serotypes are more likely to be missed. Various possible points of contamination have been identified during these investigations, including contamination during production and harvest, initial processing and packing, distribution, and final processing (Table 1.2). For example, fresh or inadequately composted manure is used sometimes, although *E. coli* O157:H7 has been shown to survive for up to 70 days in bovine feces[25]. Untreated or contaminated water seems to be a particularly likely source of contamination. Water used for spraying, washing, and maintaining the appearance of produce must be microbiologically safe. After two large outbreaks of salmonellosis were traced to imported cantaloupe, the melon industry considered a "Melon Safety Plan," focusing particularly on the chlorination of water used to wash melons and to make ice for shipping them. Although the extent to which the plan was implemented is unknown, no further large outbreaks have occurred. After two large outbreaks of salmonellosis were traced to a single tomato packer in the Southeast, an automated chlorination system was developed for the packing plant wash tank. Because tomatoes absorb water (and associated bacteria)

Table 1.1. Foodborne outbreaks traced to fresh produce 1990-1996.

Yr.	Pathogen	Vehicle	Cases (No.)	States (No.)	Source
'90	*S.* Chester	Cantaloupe	245	30	C.A.[a]
'90	*S.* Javiana	Tomatoes	174	4	U.S.[b]
'90	Hepatitis A	Strawberries	18	2	U.S.
'91	*S.* Poona	Cantaloupe	>400	23	U.S./C.A
'93	*E. coli* O157:H7	Apple cider	23	1	U.S.
'93	*S.* Montevideo	Tomatoes	84	3	U.S.
'94	*Shigella flexneri*	Scallions	72	2	C.A.
'95	*S.* Stanley	Alfalfa sprouts	242	17	N.K.[c]
'95	*S.* Hartford	Orange juice	63	21	U.S.
'95	*E. coli* O157:H7	Leaf lettuce	70	1	U.S.
'96	*E. coli* O157:H7	Leaf lettuce	49	2	U.S.
'96	Cyclospora	Raspberries	978	20	C.A.
'96	*E. coli* O157:H7	Apple juice	71	3	U.S.

[a]Central America
[b]United States
[c]Source not known

Table 1.2. Events and potential contamination sources during produce processing.

Event	Contamination sources
Production and harvest	
Growing, picking, bundling	Irrigation water, manure, lack of field sanitation
Initial processing	
Washing, waxing, sorting, boxing	Wash water, handling
Distribution	
Trucking	Ice, dirty trucks
Final processing	
Slicing, squeezing, shredding, peeling.	Wash water, handling, cross-contamination

if washed in water colder than they are, particular attention was also focused on the temperature of the water bath[26,27]. No further outbreaks have been linked to southeastern tomatoes. Similar attention is warranted for water used to rinse lettuce heads in packing sheds and to crisp them in grocery stores as well as for water used in processing other fresh produce.

A New Outbreak Scenario

Because of changes in the way food is produced and distributed, a new kind of outbreak has appeared. The traditional foodborne outbreak scenario often follows a church supper, family picnic, wedding reception, or other social event. This scenario involves an acute and highly local outbreak, with a high inoculum dose and a high attack rate. The outbreak is typically immediately apparent to those in the local group, who promptly involve medical and public health authorities. The investigation identifies a food-handling error in a small kitchen that occurs shortly before consumption. The solution is also local. Such outbreaks still occur, and handling them remains an important function of a local health department.

However, diffuse and widespread outbreaks, involving many counties, states, and even nations[28], are identified more frequently and follow an entirely different scenario. The new scenario is the result of low-level contamination of a widely distributed commercial food product. In most jurisdictions, the increase in cases may be inapparent against the background illness. The outbreak is detected only because of a fortuitous concentration of cases in one location, because the pathogen causing the outbreak is unusual, or because laboratory-based subtyping of strains collected over a wide area identifies a diffuse surge in one subtype. In such outbreaks, investigation can require coordinated efforts of a large team to clarify the extent of the outbreak, implicate a specific food, and determine the source of contamination. Often, no obvious terminal food-handling error is found. Instead, contamination is the result of an event in the industrial chain of food production. Investigating, controlling, and preventing such outbreaks can have industrywide implications.

These diffuse outbreaks can be caused by a variety of foods. Because fresh produce is usually widely distributed, most of the produce-related outbreaks listed in Table 1.1 were multistate events. Some of the largest outbreaks affected most states at once. For example, a recent outbreak of *Salmonella* Enteritidis infections caused by a nationally distributed brand of ice cream affected the entire nation[29].

Although it caused an estimated 250,000 illnesses, it was detected only when vigorous routine surveillance identified a surge in reported infections with *S*. Enteritidis in one area of southern Minnesota. The consumers affected did not make food-handling errors with their ice cream, so food safety instruction could not have prevented this outbreak. The ice cream premix was transported after pasteurization to the ice cream factory in tanker trucks that had been used to haul raw eggs. The huge epidemic was the result of a basic failure on an industrial scale to separate the raw from the cooked.

S. Enteritidis infections also illustrate why surveillance and investigation of sporadic cases are needed. A diffuse increase in sporadic cases can occur well before a local or large outbreak focuses attention on the emergence of a pathogen. The isolation rate for *S*. Enteritidis began to increase sharply in the New England region in 1978; all cases were sporadic. In 1982, an outbreak in a New England nursing home was traced to eggs from a local supplier. However, the egg connection was not really appreciated until 1986, when a large multistate outbreak of *S*. Enteritidis infections was traced to stuffed pasta made with raw eggs and labeled "fully cooked." This outbreak, affecting an estimated 3,000 persons in seven states, led to the documentation that *S*. Enteritidis was present on egg-laying farms and to the subsequent demonstration that both outbreaks and sporadic cases of infections were associated with shell eggs[19,30]. Since then, Enteritidis has become the most common serotype of Salmonella isolated in the United States, accounting for 25% of all *Salmonella* reported in the country and causing outbreaks coast to coast. Eggs remain the dominant source of these infections, causing large outbreaks when they are pooled and undercooked and individual sporadic cases among consumers who eat individual eggs[20,31]. Perhaps focused investigation and control measures taken when the localized increase in sporadic Salmonella cases was just beginning might have prevented the subsequent spread.

Changing Surveillance Strategies

In the United States, surveillance for diseases of major public health importance has been conducted for many years. The legal framework for surveillance resides in the state public health epidemiology offices, which share data with CDC. The first surveillance systems depended on physician or coroner notification of specific diseases and conditions, with reports going first to the local health department, then to state and federal offices. Now electronic, this form of surveillance is still used for many specific conditions[32]. In 1962, a second channel was developed specifically for *Salmonella*, to take advantage of the added public health information provided by subtyping the strains of bacteria[33]. Clinical laboratories that isolated *Salmonella* from humans were requested or required to send the strains to the state public health laboratory for serotyping. Although knowing the serotype is usually of little benefit to the individual patient, it has been critical to protecting and improving the health of the public at large. Serotyping allows cases that might otherwise appear unrelated to be included in an investigation because they are of the same serotype. Moreover, infections that are close in time and space to an outbreak but are caused by nonoutbreak serotypes and are probably unrelated can be discounted. Results of serotyping are now sent electronically from public health laboratories and can be rapidly analyzed and summarized. *Salmonella* serotyping was the first subtype-based surveillance system and is a model for similar systems[34]. Yet another source of surveillance data involves summary reports of foodborne disease outbreak investigations from local and state health departments[35]. About 400 such outbreaks are reported annually, by a system that remains paper-based, labor-intensive, and slow.

Existing surveillance systems provide a limited and relatively inexpensive net for tracing large-scale trends in foodborne diseases under surveillance and for detecting outbreaks of established pathogens in the United States. However, they are less sensitive to diffuse outbreaks of common pathogens, provide little detail on sporadic cases, and are not easy to extend to emerging pathogens. In the future, changes in health delivery may impinge on the way that diagnoses are made and reported, leading to artifactual changes in reported disease incidence.

Therefore, CDC, in collaboration with state health departments and federal food regulatory agencies, is enhancing national surveillance for foodborne diseases in several ways. First, the role of subtyping in public health laboratories is being expanded to encompass new molecular subtyping methods. Beginning in 1997, a national subtyping network for *E. coli* O157:H7 of participating state public health department laboratories and CDC will use a single standardized laboratory protocol to subtype strains of this important pathogen. The standard method, pulsed-field gel electrophoresis, can be easily adapted to other bacterial pathogens. In this network, each participating laboratory will be able to routinely compare the genetic gel patterns of strains of *E. coli* O157:H7 with the patterns in a national pattern bank. This will enable rapid detection of clusters of related cases within the state and will focus investigative resources on the cases most likely to be linked. It will also enable related cases scattered across several states to be linked so that a common source can be sought.

Another surveillance strategy, now implemented, is active surveillance in sentinel populations. Since January 1996, at five U.S. sentinel sites, additional surveillance resources make it possible to contact laboratories directly for regular reporting of bacterial infections likely to be foodborne[36]. In addition, surveys of the population, physicians, and laboratories measure the proportion of diarrheal diseases that are undiagnosed and unreported so that the true disease incidence can be estimated. This surveillance, known as FoodNet, is the platform on which more detailed investigations, including case-control studies of sporadic cases of common foodborne infections, are being conducted.

Yet another new surveillance initiative is the routine monitoring of antimicrobial resistance among a sample of *Salmonella* and *E. coli* O157:H7 bacteria isolated from humans[37]. A new cluster detection algorithm is being applied routinely to surveillance data for *Salmonella* at the national level, making it possible to detect and flag possible outbreaks as soon as the data are reported[38]. Implementation of such algorithms for other infections and at the state level will further increase the usefulness of routine surveillance.

Further enhancements are possible as active surveillance through FoodNet is extended to a wider spectrum of infections, including foodborne parasitic and viral infections. In 1997, active surveillance for *Cyclospora* began in FoodNet, which quickly resulted in the detection of a diffuse outbreak among persons who had been on a Caribbean cruise ship that made stops in Mexico and Central America (CDC, unpub. data). Application of standardized molecular subtyping methods to other foodborne pathogens will provide a more sensitive warning system for diffuse outbreaks of a variety of pathogens. To handle outbreaks in areas not covered by FoodNet, standard surveillance and investigative capacities in state health department epidemiology offices and laboratories should be strengthened. In addition, enhanced international consultation will be critical to better detect and investigate international or global outbreaks[28].

Implications of the New Outbreak Scenario for Public Health Activities

Our public health infrastructure is tiered, both in surveillance responsibilities and in response to emergency situations[39]. At the local level, the county or city health department, first developed in response to epidemic cholera and other challenges in the 19th century, is responsible for most basic surveillance, investigation, and prevention activities. At the state level, epidemiologists, public health laboratorians, sanitarians, and educators conduct statewide surveillance and prevention activities and consult with and support local authorities. At the national level, CDC is the primary risk-assessment agency for public health hazards and conducts the primary national surveillance as well as epidemic response in support of state health departments. The Food and Drug Administration, Department of Agriculture, and Environmental Protection Agency are the primary regulatory agencies, charged with specific responsibilities regarding the nation's food and water supplies that interlock and are not always predictable. The Food and Drug Administration regulates low-acid canned foods, imported foods, pasteurized milk, many seafoods, rabbits raised for meat, and food and water provided on aircraft and trains. The Department of Agriculture regulates meat and poultry, including primary slaughter and further processing, and pasteurized eggs; investigates animal and plant diseases; and maintains the county extension outreach program. Shell eggs do not have a clear regulatory home, as the Department of Agriculture regulates the grading of shell eggs for quality, but the Food and Drug Administration, since 1995, has responsibility for the microbiologic safety of shell eggs.

The new outbreak scenario has several implications for the practice of public health, starting at the local level. One is that when diffuse outbreaks are detected, a local health department may need to investigate a few cases that are part of a larger outbreak despite their apparently small local impact. Second, an apparently local outbreak may herald the first recognized manifestation of a national or even international event.

When a diffuse outbreak of a potentially foodborne pathogen is detected, rapid investigation is needed to determine whether the outbreak is foodborne, and if possible, identify a specific food vehicle. These investigations, which typically include case-control studies, may need to be conducted in several locations at once. While all cases or all affected states may not need to be included in such an investigation, combining cases from several locations in one investigation and repeating the investigation in more than one location can be helpful. For example, in a recent international outbreak of *Salmonella* Stanley infections traced to alfalfa sprouts, concentrations of cases in Arizona, Michigan, and Finland led to case-control studies in each location, each of which linked illness to eating sprouts grown from the same batch of alfalfa seeds. This proved that the seeds were contaminated at the source[40]. Parallel investigations can also lead to new twists. In the large West Coast outbreak of *E. coli* O157:H7 infections in 1993, a parallel investigation conducted in Nevada identified a type of hamburger other than the one implicated in the initial case-control investigation in Washington, leading to a broader recall and a more complete investigation of the circumstances of contamination[15,41]. Because well-conducted investigations may lead to major product recalls, industrial review, and overhaul, and even international embargoes, it is essential that they be of the highest scientific quality.

Foodborne outbreaks are investigated for two main reasons. The first is to identify and control an ongoing source by emergency action: product recall, restaurant closure, or other temporary but definitive solutions. The second reason is to learn how to prevent future similar outbreaks from occurring. In the long run this second purpose will have an even greater impact on public health than simply identifying and halting the outbreaks. Because all the answers are not available and existing regulations may not be sufficient to prevent outbreaks, the scientific investigation often requires a careful evaluation of the chain of production. This traceback is an integral part of the outbreak investigation. It is not a search for regulatory violations, but rather an effort to determine where and how contamination occurred. Often, the contamination scenario reveals that a critical point has been lost. Therefore, epidemiologists must participate in traceback investigations.

Intervention during outbreaks often depends on having enough good epidemiologic data to act with confidence, without waiting for a definitive laboratory test, particularly if potentially lethal illnesses are involved. For example, if five persons with classic clinical botulism ate at the same restaurant the preceding day (but have nothing else apparent in common), prudence dictates closing the restaurant quickly while the outbreak is sorted out—that is, before a specific food is identified or confirmatory cultures are made, which may take several days or even weeks. Good epidemiologic data, including evidence of a clear statistical association with a specific exposure, biologic plausibility of the illness syndrome, the potential hazard of that food, and the logical consistency of distribution of the suspect food and cases are essential.

The role of the regulatory agency laboratory is also affected by the new scenario. Because of the short shelf life and broad distribution of many of the new foods responsible for infection, by the time the outbreak is recognized and investigated the relevant food may no longer be available for culture. Because contamination may be restricted to a single production lot, blind sampling of similar foods that does not include the implicated lot can give a false sense of security. Good epidemiologic information pointing to contamination of a specific food or production lot should guide the microbiologic sampling and the interpretation of the results. Available methods may be insufficient to detect low-level contamination, even of well-established pathogens.

New Approaches to the Prevention of Foodborne Disease

Meeting the complex challenge of foodborne disease prevention will require the collaboration of regulatory agencies and industry to make food safely and keep it safe throughout the industrial chain of production. Prevention can be "built in" to the industry by identifying and controlling the key points—from field, farm, or fishing ground to the dinner table—at which contamination can either occur or be eliminated. The general strategy known as Hazard Analysis and Critical Control Points (HACCP) replaces the strategy of final product inspection. Some simple control strategies are self-evident, once the reality of microbial contamination is recognized. For example, shipping fruit from Central America with clean ice or in closed refrigerator trucks, rather than with ice made from untreated river water, is common sense. Similarly, requiring oyster harvesters to use toilets with holding tanks on their oyster boats is an obvious way to reduce fecal contamination of shallow oyster beds. Pasteurization provides the extra barrier that will prevent *E. coli* O157:H7 and other pathogens from contaminating a large batch of freshly squeezed juice.

For many foodborne diseases, multiple choices for prevention are available, and the best answer may be to apply several steps simultaneously. For *E. coli* O157:H7 infections related to the cattle reservoir, pasteurizing milk and cooking meat thoroughly provide an important measure of protection but are insufficient by themselves. Options for better control include continued improvements in slaughter plant hygiene and control measures under HACCP, developing additives to cattle feed that alter the microbial growth either in the feed or in the bovine rumen to make cows less hospitable hosts for *E. coli* O157, immunizing or otherwise protecting the cows so that they do not become infected in the first place, and irradiating beef after slaughter. For *C. jejuni* infections related to the poultry reservoir, future control options may include modification of the slaughter process to reduce contamination of chicken carcasses by bile or by water baths, freezing chicken carcasses to reduce *Campylobacter* counts, chlorinating the water that chickens drink to prevent them from getting infected, vaccinating chickens, and irradiating poultry carcasses after slaughter.

Outbreaks are often fertile sources of new research questions. Translating these questions into research agendas is an important part of the overall prevention effort. Applied research is needed to improve strategies of subtyping and surveillance. Veterinary and agricultural research on the farm is needed to answer the questions about whether and how a pathogen such as *E. coli* O157:H7 persists in the bovine reservoir, to establish the size and dynamics of a reservoir for this organism in wild deer, and to look at potential routes of contamination connecting animal manure and lettuce fields. More research is needed regarding foods defined as sources in large outbreaks to develop better control strategies and better barriers to contamination and microbial growth and to understand the behavior of new pathogens in specific foods. Research is also needed to improve the diagnosis, clinical management, and treatment of severe foodborne infections and to improve our understanding of the pathogenesis of new and emerging pathogens. To assess and evaluate potential prevention strategies, applied research is needed into the costs and potential benefits of each or of combinations.

To prepare for the 21st century, we will enhance our public health food safety infrastructure by adding new surveillance and subtyping strategies and strengthening the ability of public health practitioners to investigate and respond quickly. We need to encourage the prudent use of antibiotics in animal and human medicine to limit antimicrobial resistance. We need to continue basic and applied research into the microbes that cause foodborne disease and into the mechanisms by which they contaminate our foods and cause outbreaks and sporadic cases. Better understanding of foodborne pathogens is the foundation for new approaches to disease prevention and control.

— by Robert V. Tauxe

Address for correspondence: Centers for Disease Control and Prevention, 1600 Cliftvon Road, Atlanta, GA 30333 USA; 404-639-3311; 800-311-3435.

References

1. Blake PA, Merson MH, Weaver RE, Hollis DG, Heublein PC. Disease caused by a marine vibrio: clinical characteristics and epidemiology. *N Engl J Med* 1979;300:1-5.

2. Riley LW, Remis RS, Helgerson SD, McGee HB, Wells JG, Davis BR, et al. Hemorrhagic colitis associated with a rare *Escherichia coli* serotype. *N Engl J Med* 1983;308:681.

3. Martin ML, Shipman LD, Wells JG, Potter ME, Hedberg K, Wachsmuth IK, et al. Isolation of *Escherichia coli* O157:H7 from dairy cattle associated with two cases of hemolytic uremic syndrome. *Lancet* 1986;2:1043.

4. Ortega YR, Sterling CR, Gilman RH, Cama VA, Diaz F. *Cyclospora* species — a new protozoan pathogen of humans. *N Engl J Med* 1993;328:1308-12.

5. Herwaldt BL, Ackers M-L, the *Cyclospora* Working Group. International outbreak of cyclosporiasis associated with imported raspberries. *N Engl J Med*. In press 1997.

6. Jackson LA, Wenger JD. Listeriosis: a foodborne disease. *Infections in Medicine* 1993;10:61-6.

7. Dekeyser PJ, Gossin-Detrain M, Butzler JP, Sternon J. Acute enteritis due to related *Vibrio*; first positive stool cultures. *J Infect Dis* 1972;125:390-2.

8. Tauxe RV. Epidemiology of *Campylobacter jejuni* infections in the United States and other industrialized nations. In: *Nachamkin I*, Blaser MJ, Tompkins L, editors. *Campylobacter jejuni*: current status and future trends, eds. Washington (DC): *American Society of Microbiology*, 1992. pp 9-19.

9. Tauxe RV, Vandepitte J, Wauters G, Martin SM, Goosens V, DeMol P, et al. *Yersinia enterocolitica* infections and pork: the missing link. *Lancet* 1987;1:1129-32.

10. World Health Organization. Worldwide spread of infections with *Yersinia enterocolitica*. *WHO Chronicle* 1976;30:494-6.

11. Rodrigue DC, Tauxe RV, Rowe B. International increase in *Salmonella enteritidis*: a new pandemic? *Epidemiol Infect* 1990;105:21-7.

12. Centers for Disease Control and Prevention. Multidrug-resistant *Salmonella serotype Typhimurium* — United States, 1996. *MMWR Morb Mortal Wkly Rep* 1997;46:308-10.

13. Endt HP, Ruijs GJ, van Klingeren B, Jansen WH, van der Reyden T, Mouton RP. Quinolone resistance in *Campylobacter* isolated from man and poultry following the introduction of fluoroquinolones in veterinary medicine. *J Antimicrob Chemother* 1991;27:199-208.

14. Lee LA, Puhr ND, Maloney K, Bean NH, Tauxe RV. Increase in antimicrobial-resistant *Salmonella* infections in the United States, 1989-1990. *J Infect Dis* 1994;170:128-34.

15. Cieslak PR, Noble SJ, Maxson DJ, Empey LC, Ravenholt O, Legarza G, et al. Hamburger-associated *Escherichia coli* O157:H7 in Las Vegas: a hidden epidemic. *Am J Public Health* 1997;87:176-80.

16. Humphrey TJ, Greenwood M, Gilbert RJ, Rowe B, Chapman PA. The survival of salmonellas in shell eggs cooked under simulated domestic conditions. *Epidemiol Infect* 1989;103:35-45.

17. Kirkland KB, Meriwether RA, Leiss JK, MacKenzie WR. Steaming oysters does not prevent Norwalk-like gastroenteritis. *Public Health Rep* 1996;111:527-30.

18. Holmberg SD, Feldman RA. New and newer enteric pathogens: stages in our knowledge. *Am J Public Health* 1984;74:205-7.

19. St. Louis ME, Morse DL, Potter ME, DeMelfi TM, Guzewich JJ, Tauxe RV, et al. The emergence of Grade A eggs as a major source of *Salmonella enteritidis* infections: implications for the control of salmonellosis. *JAMA* 1988;259:2103-7.

20. Mishu B, J Koehler, Lee LA, Rodrigue D, Brenner FH, Blake P, Tauxe RV. Outbreaks of *Salmonella enteritidis* infections in the United States, 1985-1991. *J Infect Dis* 1994;169:547-52.

21. Besser RE, Lett SM, Weber JT, Doyle MP, Barrett TJ, Wells JG, Griffin PM. An outbreak of diarrhea and hemolytic uremic syndrome from *Escherichia coli* O157:H7 in fresh-pressed apple cider. *JAMA* 1993;269:2217-20.

22. Keene WE, Sazie E, Kok J, Rice DH, Hancock DD, Balan VK, et al. An outbreak of *Escherichia coli* O157:H7 infections traced to jerky made from deer meat. *JAMA* 1997;277:1229-31.

23. Kohn MA, Farley TA, Ando T, Curtis M, Wilson SA, Jin Q, et al. An outbreak of Norwalk virus gastroenteritis associated with eating raw oysters: implications for maintaining safe oyster beds. *JAMA* 1995;273:466-71.

24. Tauxe R, Kruse H, Hedberg C, Potter M, Madden J, Wachsmuth K. Microbial hazards and emerging issues associated with produce; a preliminary report to the National Advisory Committee on Microbiologic Criteria for Foods. *Journal of Food Protection*. In press 1997.

25. Wang G, Zhao T, Doyle MP. Fate of enterohemorrhagic *Escherichia coli* O157:H7 in bovine feces. *Appl Environ Microbiol* 1996;62:2567-70.

26. Zhuang R-Y, Beuchat LR, Angulo FJ. Fate of *Salmonella montevideo* on and in raw tomatoes as affected by temperature and treatment with chlorine. *Appl Environ Microbiol* 1995;61:2127-31.

27. Rushing JW, Angulo FJ, Beuchat LR. Implementation of a HACCP program in a commercial fresh-market tomato packinghouse: a model for the industry. *Dairy, Food and Environmental Sanitation* 1996;16:549-53.

28. Tauxe RV, Hughes JM. International investigations of outbreaks of foodborne disease: public health responds to the globalization of food. *BMJ* 1996;313:1093-4.

29. Hennessey TW, Hedberg CW, Slutsker L, White KE, Besser-Wiek JM, Moen ME, et al. A national outbreak of *Salmonella enteritidis* infections from ice cream. *N Engl J Med* 1996;334:1281-6.

30. Passarro DJ, Reporter R, Mascola L, Kilman L, Malcolm GB, Rolka H, et al. Epidemic *Salmonella Enteritidis* infection in Los Angeles County, California: the predominance of phage type 4. *West J Med* 1996;165:126-30.

31. Centers for Disease Control and Prevention. Outbreaks of *Salmonella* serotype Enteritidis infection associated with consumption of raw shell eggs—United States, 1994-1995. *MMWR Morb Mortal Wkly Rep* 1996;45:737-42.

32. Centers for Disease Control and Prevention. Summary of notifiable diseases, United States, 1995. *MMWR Morb Mortal Wkly Rep* 1995;44(53).

33. Centers for Disease Control and Prevention. Proceedings of a national conference on salmonellosis, March 11-13, 1964. U.S. Public Health Service Publication No 1262. Washington (DC): U.S. Government Printing Office; 1965.

34. Bean NH, Morris SM, Bradford H. PHLIS: an electronic system for reporting public health data from remote sites. *Am J Public Health* 1992;82:1273-6.

35. Bean NH, Goulding JS, Lao C, Angulo FJ. Surveillance for foodborne-disease outbreaks United States, 1988-1992. *CDC Surveillance Summaries*, October 25, 1996. *MMWR Morb Mortal Wkly Rep* 1996;45(SS-5).

36. Centers for Disease Control and Prevention. Foodborne Diseases Active Surveillance Network, 1996. *MMWR Morb Mortal Wkly Rep* 1997;46:258-61.

37. Centers for Disease Control and Prevention. Establishment of a national surveillance program for antimicrobial resistance in *Salmonella*. *MMWR Morb Mortal Wkly Rep* 1996;45:110-1.

38. Hutwagner LC, Maloney EK, Bean NH, Slutsker L, Martin SM. Using laboratory-based surveillance data for prevention: an algorithm for detecting *Salmonella* outbreaks. *Emerg Infect Dis* 1997;3:395-400.

39. Meriwether RA. Blueprint for a national public health surveillance system for the 21st Century. *Journal of Public Health Management and Practice* 1996;2:16-23.

40. Mahon BE, Pönkä A, Hall WN, Komatsu K, Dietrich SE, Siitonen A, et al. An international outbreak of *Salmonella* infections caused by alfalfa sprouts grown from contaminated seed. *J Infect Dis* 1997;175:876-82.

41. Bell BP, Goldoft M, Griffin PM, Davis MA, Gordon DC, Tarr PI, et al. A multistate outbreak of *Escherichia coli* O157:H7-associated bloody diarrhea and hemolytic uremic syndrome from hamburgers: the Washington experience. *JAMA* 1994;272:1349-53.

Chapter 2

A Guide to Safe Food Handling

This chapter tells you what to do at each step in food handling—from shopping through storing leftovers—to avoid food poisoning.

Never had food poisoning? Actually, it's called foodborne illness. Perhaps you have, but thought you were sick with the flu. Some 33 million Americans could suffer from foodborne illness this year.

Why? Because under the right conditions, bacteria you can't see, smell or taste can make you sick.

It doesn't have to happen, though. Many such cases could be avoided if people just handled food properly. So here's what to do...

When You Shop—
Buy Cold Food Last, Get it Home Fast

- When you're out, grocery shop last. Take food straight home to the refrigerator. Never leave food in a hot car!

- Don't buy anything you won't use before the use-by date.

- Don't buy food in poor condition. Make sure refrigerated food is cold to the touch. Frozen food should be rock-solid. Canned goods should be free of dents, cracks or bulging lids, which can indicate a serious food poisoning threat.

Home and Garden Bulletin, No. 248, revised October 1995; U.S. Department of Agriculture; Food Safety and Inspection Service.

When You Store Food—Keep it Safe, Refrigerate

Check the temperature of your refrigerator with an appliance thermometer. To keep bacteria in check, the refrigerator should run at 40° F; the freezer unit at 0° F. Keep your refrigerator as cold as possible without freezing milk or lettuce.

- Freeze fresh meat, poultry or fish immediately if you can't use it within a few days.

- Put packages of raw meat, poultry or fish on a plate before refrigerating so their juices won't drip on other food. Raw juices often contain bacteria.

When You Prepare Food—Keep Everything Clean, Thaw in Refrigerator

- Wash hands in hot soapy water before preparing food and after using the bathroom, changing diapers and handling pets.

- Harmful bacteria multiply quickly in kitchen towels, sponges and cloths. Wash cloth items often in hot-cycle in your machine. Consider using paper towels to clean up meat and poultry juices. Avoid sponges or place them in the dishwasher daily to kill bacteria.

- Keep raw meat, poultry and fish and their juices away from other food. For instance, wash your hands, cutting board, knife and countertops in hot soapy water after cutting up the chicken and before slicing salad ingredients. Also use hot soapy water to wash sink and kitchen faucet handles the raw meat or your "meat-covered" hands have touched.

- Use plastic or other non-porous cutting boards rather than wooden ones. These boards should be run through the dishwasher after use.

- **What about antibacterial sanitizers in the kitchen?** Food handling experts feel hot soapy water used properly should protect you adequately against foodborne bacteria. However, kitchen sanitizers (including a mixture of bleach and water) can provide some added protection. NOTE: Sanitizer product directions must be followed carefully as products differ greatly.

- Thaw frozen food in the refrigerator or in the microwave, NOT on the kitchen counter. Marinate in the refrigerator too.

When You're Cooking—Cook Thoroughly

It takes thorough cooking to kill harmful bacteria, so you're taking chances when you eat meat, poultry, fish or eggs that are raw or only partly cooked. Plus, hamburger that is red in the middle and rare steak and roast beef are also undercooked from the safety standpoint.

- Generally cook red meat to 160° F. Cook poultry to 180° F. Use a meat thermometer to check that it's cooked all the way through.

- To check visually, red meat is done when it's brown or gray inside. Poultry juices run clear. Fish flakes with a fork.

- Ground meat, where bacteria can spread throughout the meat during processing, should be cooked to at least 160° F. This means there is no pink left in the middle or in juices. You can allow large cuts like roasts to stay slightly pink in the center as long as they've reached at least 140° F (medium-rare). Do not serve any cut at this low temperature if you have scored (cut or poked with a fork) or tenderized it before cooking, thus forcing surface bacteria into the center.

- *Salmonella*, a bacteria that causes food poisoning, can grow inside fresh, unbroken eggs. So cook eggs until the yolk and white are firm, not runny. Scramble eggs to a firm texture. Don't use recipes in which eggs remain raw or only partially cooked.

Safe Microwaving

A great timesaver, the microwave has one food safety disadvantage. It sometimes leaves cold spots in food. Bacteria can survive in these spots. So...

- Cover food with a lid or plastic wrap so steam can aid thorough cooking. Vent wrap and make sure it doesn't touch the food.

- Stir and rotate your food for even cooking. No turntable? Rotate the dish by hand once or twice during cooking.

- Observe the standing time called for in a recipe or package directions. During the standing time, food finishes cooking.

- Use the oven temperature probe or a meat thermometer to check that food is done. Insert it at several spots.

When You Serve Food—Never Leave it Out Over 2 Hours

- Use clean dishes and utensils to serve food, not those used in preparation. Serve grilled food on a clean plate too, not one that held raw meat, poultry or fish.

- Never leave perishable food out of the refrigerator over 2 hours! Bacteria that can cause food poisoning grow quickly at warm temperatures.

- Pack lunches in insulated carriers with a cold pack. Caution children never to leave lunches in direct sun or on a warm radiator.

- Carry picnic food in a cooler with a cold pack. When possible, put the cooler in the shade. Keep the lid on as much as you can.

- Party time? Keep cold party food on ice or serve it throughout the gathering from platters from the refrigerator.

Likewise, divide hot party food into smaller serving platters. Keep platters refrigerated until time to warm them up for serving.

When You Handle Leftovers—Use Small Containers for Quick Cooling

- Divide large amounts of leftovers into small, shallow containers for quick cooling in the refrigerator. Don't pack the refrigerator—cool air must circulate to keep food safe.

- With poultry or other stuffed meats, remove stuffing and refrigerate it in separate containers.

Reheating

- Bring sauces, soups and gravy to a boil. Heat other leftovers thoroughly to 165° F.

- Microwave leftovers using a lid or vented plastic wrap for thorough heating.

Kept It Too Long?—When in Doubt, Throw It Out

Safe refrigerator and freezer storage time limits are given for many common foods in the "Cold Storage" table in this chapter. But what about something you totally forgot about and may have kept too long?

- *Danger*—never taste food that looks or smells strange to see if you can still use it. Just discard it.

- Is it moldy? The mold you see is only the tip of the iceberg. The poisons molds can form are found under the surface of the food. So, while you can sometimes save hard cheese and salamis and firm fruits and vegetables by cutting the mold out—remove a large area around it, most moldy food should be discarded.

Power's Out—Your Freezer

Without power, a full upright or chest freezer will keep everything frozen for about 2 days. A half-full freezer will keep food frozen 1 day.

If power will be coming back on fairly soon, you can make the food last longer by keeping the door shut as much as possible.

If power will be off for an extended period, take food to friends' freezers, locate a commercial freezer or use dry ice.

Your Refrigerator-Freezer Combination

Without power, the refrigerator section will keep food cool 4-6 hours depending on the kitchen temperature.

A full, well-functioning freezer unit should keep food frozen for 2 days. A half-full freezer unit should keep things frozen about 1 day.

Block ice can keep food on the refrigerator shelves cooler. Dry ice can be added to the freezer unit. You can't touch dry ice and you shouldn't breathe the fumes, so follow handling instructions carefully.

Thawed Food?

Food still containing ice crystals or that feels refrigerator-cold can be refrozen.

Discard any thawed food that has risen to room temperature and remained there 2 hours or more. Immediately discard anything with a strange color or odor.

Table 2.1a. Cold Storage (continued on next page)

NOTE: These SHORT but safe time limits will help keep refrigerated food from spoiling or becoming dangerous to eat These time limits will keep frozen food at top quality.

Product	Refrigerator (40° F)	Freezer (0° F)
Eggs		
Fresh, in shell	3 weeks	Don't freeze
Raw yolks, whites	2-4 days	1 year
Hardcooked	1 week	Don't freeze well
Liquid pasteurized eggs or		
egg substitutes, opened	3 days	Don't freeze
unopened	10 days	1 year
Mayonnaise, commercial		
Refrigerate after opening	2 months	Don't freeze
TV Dinners, Frozen Casseroles		
Keep frozen until ready to serve		3-4 months
Deli & Vacuum-Packed Products		
Store-prepared (or homemade)		
egg, chicken, tuna, ham,		
macaroni salads	3-5 days	Deli and vacuum-
Pre-stuffed pork & lamb chops,		packed products
chicken breasts stuffed with		don't freeze well
dressing	1 day	
Store-cooked convenience meals	1-2 days	
Commercial brand vacuum-		
packed dinners with USDA seal	2 weeks, unopened	
Soups & Stews		
Vegetable or meat-added	3-4 days	2-3 months
Hamburger, Ground & Stew Meats		
Hamburger & stew meats	1-2 days	3-4 months
Ground turkey, veal, pork,		
lamb & mixtures of them	1-2 days	3-4 months
Hotdogs & Lunch Meats		
Hotdogs, opened package	1 week	
unopened package	2 weeks	In freezer wrap,
Lunch meats, opened	3-5 days	1-2 months
unopened	2 weeks	

Table 2.1b. Cold Storage (continued from previous page).

Product	Refrigerator (40° F)	Freezer (0° F)
Bacon & Sausage		
Bacon	7 days	1 month
Sausage, raw from pork, beef, turkey	1-2 days	1-2 months
Smoked breakfast links, patties	7 days	1-2 months
Hard sausage-pepperoni, jerky sticks	2-3 weeks	1-2 months
Ham, Corned Beef		
Corned beef		Drained, wrapped
in pouch with pickling juices	5-7 days	1 month
Ham, canned,		
Label says keep refrigerated	6-9 months	Don't freeze
Ham, fully cooked—whole	7 days	1-2 months
Ham, fully cooked—half	3-5 days	1-2 months
Ham, fully cooked—slices	3-4 days	1-2 months
Fresh Meat		
Steaks, beef	3-5 days	6-12 months
Chops, pork	3-5 days	4-6 months
Chops, lamb	3-5 days	6-9 months
Roasts, beef	3-5 days	6-12 months
Roasts, lamb	3-5 days	6-9 months
Roasts, pork & veal	3-5 days	4-6 months
Variety meats—Tongue,		
brain, kidneys, liver, heart,		
chitterlings	1-2 days	3-4 months
Meat Leftovers		
Cooked meat and		
meat dishesv3-4 days	2-3 months	
Gravy and meat broth	1-2 days	2-3 months
Fresh Poultry		
Chicken or turkey, whole	1-2 days	1 year
Chicken or turkey pieces	1-2 days	9 months
Giblets	1-2 days	3-4 months
Cooked Poultry, Leftover		
Fried chicken	3-4 days	4 months
Cooked poultry dishes	3-4 days	4-6 months
Pieces, plain	3-4 days	4 months
Pieces covered with broth, gravy	1-2 days	6 months
Chicken nuggets, patties	1-2 days	1-3 months

Table 2.2. Cooking Temperatures

Product	Fahrenheit
Eggs & Egg Dishes	
Eggs	Cook until yolk & white are firm
Egg dishes	160
Ground Meat & Meat Mixtures	
Turkey, chicken	165
Veal, beef, lamb, pork	160
Fresh Beef	
Medium Rare	145
Medium	160
Well Done	170
Fresh Veal	
Medium Rare	145
Medium	160
Well Done	170
Fresh Lamb	
Medium Rare	145
Medium	160
Well Done	170
Fresh Pork	
Medium	160
Well Done	170
Poultry	
Chicken, whole	180
Turkey, whole	180
Poultry breasts, roasts	170
Poultry thighs, wings	Cook until juices run clear
Stuffing (cooked alone or in bird)	165
Duck & Goose	180
Ham	
Fresh (raw)	160
Pre-cooked (to reheat)	140

Is It Food Poisoning?

If you or a family member develop nausea, vomiting, diarrhea, fever or cramps, you could have food poisoning. Unfortunately, it's not always easy to tell since, depending on the illness, symptoms can appear anywhere from 30 minutes to 2 weeks after eating bad food. Most often, though, people get sick within 4 to 48 hours after eating.

In more serious cases, food poisoning victims may have nervous system problems like paralysis, double vision or trouble swallowing or breathing.

If symptoms are severe or the victim is very young, old, pregnant, or already ill, call a doctor or go to the hospital right away.

When to Report Foodborne Illness

You or your physician should report serious cases of foodborne illness to the local health department. Report any food poisoning incidents if the food involved came from a restaurant or commercial outlet.

Give a detailed, but short account of the incident. If the food is a commercial product, have it in hand so you can describe it over the phone.

If you're asked to keep the food refrigerated so officials can examine it later, follow directions carefully.

For more information on food handling, call:
USDA's Meat and Poultry Hotline
1-800-535-4555
10-4 weekdays Eastern Time

Chapter 3

The Color of Meat and Poultry

I've just opened a package of fresh chicken and the skin looks blue. Is it safe to use?

My package of ground beef is dark in the center. Is this old meat?

The turkey was cooked according to the directions, but the breast meat is pink. Will it make us sick?

These are just a few of the many questions received at the U.S. Department of Agriculture's Meat and Poultry Hotline concerning the color of meat and poultry. Color is important when meat and poultry are purchased, stored, and cooked. Often an attractive, bright color is a consideration for the purchase. So, why are there differences in the color and what do they mean? Listed below are some questions and answers to help you understand the color differences.

1. What factors affect the color of meat and poultry?

Myoglobin, a protein, is responsible for the majority of the red color. Myoglobin doesn't circulate in the blood but is fixed in the tissue cells and is purplish in color. When it is mixed with oxygen, it becomes oxymyoglobin and produces a bright red color. The remaining color comes from the hemoglobin, which occurs mainly in the circulating blood, but a small amount can be found in the tissues after slaughter.

Food Safety and Inspection Service; United States Department of Agriculture, Washington, D.C. 20250-3700, July 1998.

33

Color is also influenced by the age of the animal, the species, sex, diet, and even the exercise it gets. The meat from older animals will be darker in color because the myoglobin level increases with age. Exercised muscles are always darker in color, which means the same animal can have variations of color in its muscles.

In addition, the color of meat and poultry can change as it is being stored at retail and in the home (see explanation in question 5). When safely stored in the refrigerator or freezer, color changes are normal for fresh meat and poultry.

2. Does a change in color indicate spoilage?

Change in color alone does not mean the product is spoiled. Color changes are normal for fresh product. With spoilage there can be a change in color—often a fading or darkening. In addition to the color change, the meat or poultry will have an off odor, be sticky or tacky to the touch, or it may be slimy. If meat has developed these characteristics, it should not be used.

3.If the color of meat and poultry changes while frozen, is it safe?

Color changes, while meat and poultry are frozen, occur just as they do in the refrigerator. Fading and darkening, for example, do not affect their safety. These changes are minimized by using freezer-type wrapping and by expelling as much air as possible from the package.

4. What are the white dried patches on frozen meat and poultry?

The white dried patches indicate freezer burn. When meat and poultry have been frozen for an extended period of time or have not been·wrapped and sealed properly, this will occur. The product remains safe to eat, but the areas with freezer burn will be dried out and tasteless and can be trimmed away if desired.

5. When displayed at the grocery store, why is some meat bright red and other meat very dark in color?

Optimum surface color of fresh meat (i.e., cherry-red for beef; dark cherry-red for lamb; grayish-pink for pork; and pale pink for veal) is highly unstable and short-lived. When meat is fresh and protected from contact with air (such as in vacuum packages), it has the purple-red color that comes from myoglobin, one of the two key pigments responsible for the color of meat. When exposed to air, myoglobin forms the pigment, oxymyoglobin, which gives meat a pleasingly cherry-red color. The use of a plastic wrap that allows oxygen to pass through it helps ensure that the cut meats will retain this bright red color. However, exposure to store lighting as well as the continued contact of myoglobin and oxymyoglobin with oxygen leads to the formation of metmyoglobin, a pigment that turns meat brownish-red. This color change alone does not mean the product is spoiled (see explanation in question 2).

6. Why is pre-packaged ground beef red on the outside and sometimes grayish-brown on the inside?

These color differences do not indicate that the meat is spoiled or old. As discussed earlier, fresh cut meat is purplish in color. Oxygen from the air reacts with meat pigments to form a bright red color which is usually seen on the surface of ground beef purchased in the supermarket. The interior of the meat may be grayish-brown due to the lack of oxygen penetrating below the surface.

7. A beef roast has darkened in the refrigerator, is it safe?

Yes, it is safe. The darkening is due to oxidation, the chemical changes in myoglobin due to the oxygen content. This is a normal change during refrigerator storage.

8. Can cooked ground beef still be pink inside?

Yes, ground beef can be pink inside after it is safely cooked. The pink color can be due to a reaction between the oven heat and myoglobin, which causes a red or pink color. It can also occur when vegetables containing nitrites are cooked along with the meat. Because doneness and safety cannot be judged by color, it is very important to use a meat thermometer when cooking ground beef. To be sure all harmful bacteria are destroyed, cook all ground beef products to an internal temperature of 160 ° F throughout.

9. What causes iridescent colors on meats?

Meat contains iron, fat, and other compounds. When light hits a slice of meat, it splits into colors like a rainbow. There are various pigments in meat compounds that can give it an iridescent or greenish cast when exposed to heat and processing. Wrapping the meat in airtight packages and storing it away from light will help prevent this situation. Iridescence does not represent decreased quality or safety of the meat.

10. What causes grayish or green color on cured meats?

Exposure to light and oxygen causes oxidation to take place, which causes the breaking down of color pigments formed during the curing process. Chemicals in the cure and oxygen, as well as energy from ultraviolet and visible light, contribute to both the chemical breakdown and microbial spoilage of the product. Cure, such as nitrite, chemically changes the color of muscle. Curing solutions are colored in order to distinguish them from other ingredients (such as sugar or salt) used in fresh and cured meat products. For example, cured raw pork is gray, but cured cooked pork (e.g., ham) is light pink.

11. What is the usual color of raw poultry?

Raw poultry can vary from a bluish-white to yellow. All of these colors are normal and are a direct result of breed, exercise, age, and/or diet. Younger poultry has less fat under the skin, which can cause the bluish cast, and the yellow skin could be a result of marigolds in the feed.

12. What causes the differences in color of raw ground poultry?

Ground poultry varies in color according to the part being ground. Darker pink means more dark meat was used and a lighter pink means more white meat was included (or skin was included). Ground poultry can contain only muscle meat and skin with attached fat in proportion to the whole bird.

13. What causes dark bones in cooked poultry?

Darkening of bones and meat around the bones occurs primarily in young (6-8 weeks) broiler-fryer chickens. Since the bones have not calcified or hardened completely, pigment from the bone marrow seeps through the bones and into the surrounding area. Freezing can also contribute to this darkening. This is an aesthetic issue and not a safety one. The meat is safe to eat when all parts have reached at least 160° F.

14. What color is safely cooked poultry?

Safely cooked poultry can vary in color from white to pink to tan. When the temperature of the poultry as measured in the thigh has reached 180° F, there is usually no other site in the bird lower than the safe temperature of 160° F. Check the temperature in several locations, being sure to include the wing joint. All the meat—including any that remains pink—is safe to eat as soon as all parts reach at least 160° F.

15. Why is some cooked poultry pink?

Chemical changes occur during cooking. Oven gases in a heated gas or electric oven react chemically with hemoglobin in the meat tissues to give it a pink tinge. Often meat of younger birds shows the most pink because their thinner skins permit oven gases to reach the flesh. Older animals have a fat layer under their skin, giving the flesh-added protection from the gases. Older poultry may be pink in spots where fat is absent from the skin. Also, nitrates and nitrites, which are often used as preservatives or may occur naturally in the feed or water supply used, can cause a pink color.

16. If fully cooked smoked poultry is pink, is it safe?

Poultry grilled or smoked outdoors can be pink, even when all parts have attained temperatures well above 160° F. There may be a pink-colored rim about one-half inch wide around the outside of the cooked product. Commercially prepared, smoked poultry is usually pink because it is prepared with natural smoke and liquid smoke flavor. Federal regulations require all processed poultry to be cooked to at least 160° F instantly, or to an equivalent level of safety attained by this minimum temperature requirement.

For additional food safety information about meat, poultry, or eggs, call the toll-free USDA Meat and Poultry Hotline at 1 (800) 535-4555; Washington, DC (202) 720-3333; TTY: 1 (800) 256-7072. It is staffed by home economists, dietitians, and food technologists weekdays from 10 a.m. to 4 p.m. Eastern time, year round. An extensive selection of food safety recordings can be heard 24 hours a day using a touch-tone phone.

Information is also available from the FSIS Web site: http://www.fsis.usda.gov

For Further Information Contact:

FSIS Food Safety Education and Communications Staff
Meat and Poultry Hotline:
1-800-535-4555 (Tollfree Nationwide)
(202) 720-3333 (Washington, DC area)
1-800-256-7072 (TDD/TTY)

Chapter 4

Critical Steps toward Safer Seafood

A tender tuna steak lightly seasoned with lemon pepper and grilled over a charcoal fire is one way to please a seafood lover's palate. Stuffed flounder, lobster thermidor, and shrimp scampi are others.

But blue marlin served up with a dose of scombroid poisoning or steamed oysters with a touch of Norwalk-like virus are more likely to turn the stomach, instead of treating the palate.

Earlier this year, 26 employees of the World Bank headquarters in Washington, D.C., developed headaches, dizziness, nausea, and rashes several hours after eating blue marlin served in their workplace cafeteria. An emergency room doctor who treated some of the victims attributed the illness to scombroid poisoning, which is caused by a toxin produced when certain fish spoil.

In 1995, the national Centers for Disease Control and Prevention reported 34 incidences of food poisoning in people who had eaten oysters harvested from certain southern U.S. waters. Health experts blamed the flu-like illness on a virus similar to the Norwalk virus, which is usually introduced into fishing areas by human sewage.

Generally, seafood is very safe to eat, says Phillip Spiller, director of the Food and Drug Administration's Office of Seafood. "On a pound-for-pound basis, seafood is as safe as, if not more safe than, other meat sources. But no food is completely safe, and problems do occur."

FDA Consumer, November-December 1997; U. S. Food and Drug Administration.

Seafood—the most perishable of flesh foods, according to FDA—comes to this country from all over the world, often traveling long distances before being processed, sold or eaten.

Spiller points out that while FDA has regulated seafood for decades, a new FDA program that goes into effect in December 1997 aims to further ensure seafood's safety. This program requires seafood processors, repackers and warehouses—both domestic and foreign exporters to this country—to follow a modern food safety system known as Hazard Analysis and Critical Control Point, or HACCP (pronounced hassip). This system focuses on identifying and preventing hazards that could cause food-borne illnesses rather than relying on spot-checks of manufacturing processes and random sampling of finished seafood products to ensure safety.

This is the first time that the HACCP system will be required for the processing and storage of a U.S. food commodity on an industry-wide basis.

Seafood safety could be further ensured if seafood retailers integrate HACCP in their operations. Although seafood retailers are exempt from the HACCP regulations, FDA, through its 1997 edition of the Food Code, encourages retailers to apply HACCP-based food safety principles, along with other recommended practices. The Food Code serves as model legislation for state and territorial agencies that license and inspect food service establishments, food vending operations, and food stores.

These efforts will be accompanied by seafood safety programs already in place, such as ongoing research by FDA's seafood safety experts and others, and the National Oceanic and Atmospheric Administration's voluntary fee-for-service inspection program.

Consumers are expected to continue their role, too, choosing seafood retailers and products carefully, and handling and serving their products with care in the home.

"Consumers are a step along the way to ensuring that only safe seafood goes in the mouth," says Mary Snyder, director of programs and enforcement policy in FDA's Office of Seafood. "They have to know what they're doing."

Reducing Hazards with HACCP

Seafood can be exposed to a range of hazards from the water to the table. Some of these hazards are natural to seafood's environment; others are introduced by humans. The hazards can involve bacteria, viruses, parasites, natural toxins, and chemical contaminants.

The HACCP system that seafood companies will have to consider and, in most cases, establish will help weed out seafood hazards with the following seven steps:

- Analyze hazards. Every processor must determine the potential hazards associated with each of its seafood products and the measures needed to control those hazards. The hazard could be biological, such as a microbe; chemical, such as mercury or a toxin; or physical, such as ground glass.

- Identify critical control points, such as cooking or cooling, where the potential hazard can be controlled or eliminated.

- Establish preventive measures with critical limits for each control point.

- Establish procedures to monitor the critical control points. This might include determining how cooking time and temperatures will be monitored and by whom.

- Establish corrective actions to take when monitoring shows that a critical limit has not been met. Such actions might include reprocessing the seafood product or disposing of it altogether.

- Establish procedures to verify that the system is working properly.

- Establish effective recordkeeping.

Also, under FDA's HACCP regulations, seafood companies will have to write and follow basic sanitation standards that ensure, for example, the use of safe water in food preparation; cleanliness of food contact surfaces, such as tables, utensils, gloves and employees' clothes; prevention of cross-contamination; and proper maintenance of hand-washing, hand-sanitizing, and toilet facilities.

In addition, molluscan shellfish handlers must follow a few additional rules; for example, they must obtain shellfish only from approved waters and only if they are properly tagged, which indicates that they have come from an approved source.

FDA estimates that more than half of the seafood eaten in this country is imported from almost 135 countries. The agency is requiring for the first time that seafood importers take certain steps to verify that their overseas' suppliers are providing seafood processed under HACCP. Food companies in some foreign countries, such as those in the European Union and in Canada, already follow HACCP, as mandated by national law. Also, FDA is working on international agreements with other countries to ensure that products imported and exported between the United States and another country are processed and inspected under a HACCP-based program.

As in the past, FDA will periodically inspect seafood processors and warehouses. But unlike in the past, when FDA's inspection reports were based mainly on activities observed during the day or days of the inspection, the required HACCP records will enable the agency to determine how well a company is complying over time.

The safety features of FDA's HACCP regulations are already incorporated into the National Seafood Inspection Program of the Department of Commerce's National Oceanic and Atmospheric Administration. For a fee, NOAA inspects seafood processors and others, checking vessels and plants for sanitation and examining products for quality. The agency certifies seafood plants that meet federal standards and rates products with grades based on their quality. Seafood processors in good standing with the program are free to use official marks on products that indicate the seafood has been federally inspected.

Additional Protections

FDA promotes seafood safety in other ways, including:

- Setting standards for seafood contaminants. FDA has established a legally binding safety limit for polychlorinated biphenyls and guidelines for safety limits for six pesticides, mercury, paralytic shellfish poison, and histamine in canned tuna. (Histamine is the chemical responsible for scombroid poisoning.)

- Administering the National Shellfish Sanitation Program, which involves 23 shellfish-producing states, plus a few non-shellfish-producing states, and nine countries. The program exercises control over all sanitation related to the growing, harvesting, shucking, packing, and interstate transportation of oysters, clams and other molluscan shellfish.

- Lending its expertise to the Interstate Shellfish Sanitation Conference, an organization of federal and state agencies and members of the shellfish industry. The conference develops uniform guidelines and procedures for state agencies that monitor shellfish safety.

- Entering into cooperative programs with states to provide training to state and local health officials who inspect fishing areas (for example, shellfish beds), seafood processing plants and warehouses, and restaurants and other retail places.

- Working with NOAA to close federal waters to fishing whenever oil spills, toxic blooms, or other phenomena threaten seafood safety.

- Sampling and analyzing fish and fishery products for toxins, chemicals and other hazards in agency laboratories.

FDA also does extensive seafood safety research at its Gulf Coast Seafood Laboratory at Dauphin Island, Ala., and its seafood laboratories in Bothell, Wash., and Washington, D.C. In addition, research at other sites around the country will be transferred early in 1998 to the agency's national seafood safety center—a joint venture with the University of Maryland's Center of Marine Biotechnology—in Columbus Center in downtown Baltimore.

The agency's seafood scientists are tackling a number of research projects, according to George Hoskin, Ph.D., director of science and applied technology in FDA's Office of Seafood:

- Identifying a legally binding action level for histamine in fish to protect consumers from scombroid poisoning.

- Developing chemical indicators for detecting decomposed fish. Decomposition is now identified by organoleptic techniques, in which highly trained people use their sense of smell and sight to determine quality. Hoskin says that chemical indicators could help reduce costs of training people in this highly skilled area and provide a quantitative rather than a qualitative measure of decomposition. "Once you've trained an organoleptic analyst, the technique is a fast, efficient way to detect decomposed fish," he says. "But a chemical indicator will make people think the measure is more objective."

- Pinpointing physiological changes that put people at risk for infection with Vibrio vulnificus, the leading cause of seafood death, so that health officials can better advise at-risk people.

- Developing cheaper and easier tests for detecting ciguatera toxin, which affects certain warm-water reef fish. Current laboratory methods are expensive and complex, Hoskin says.

A Safe Seafood Supply

A walk through just about any seafood market or through any grocery store's seafood section will show the diversity of today's U.S. seafood supply. There are crabs and clams, bass, red snapper, catfish, octopus and squid, mackerel and salmon, and many more—from throughout the country and the world. The selection is a seafood gourmet's delight.

But delight can quickly turn to disaster if the seafood is unsafe. The establishment of HACCP in the seafood industry, along with ongoing research and other federal and state activities, and careful handling by consumers, can help ensure that seafood is not only tasty and healthful but safe to eat, as well.

How to Spot a Safe Seafood Seller

Anyone who's ever smelled rotting seafood at the fish counter has a pretty good idea of what a poorly run seafood market smells like. But the absence of any strong odor doesn't necessarily mean that the seller is practicing safe food handling techniques.

Based on FDA's Food Code, here are some other points to consider:

• Employees should be in clean clothing but no outerwear and wearing hair coverings.

• They shouldn't be smoking, eating, or playing with their hair. They shouldn't be sick or have any open wounds.

• Employees should be wearing disposable gloves when handling food and change gloves after doing nonfood tasks and after handling any raw seafood.

• Fish should be displayed on a thick bed of fresh, not melting ice, preferably in a case or under some type of cover. Fish should be arranged with the bellies down so that the melting ice drains away from the fish, thus reducing the chances of spoilage.

• What's your general impression of the facility? Does it look clean? Smell clean? Is it free of flies and bugs? A well-maintained facility can indicate that the vendor is following good sanitation practices.

- Is the seafood employee knowledgeable about different types of seafood? Can he or she tell you how old the products are and explain why their seafood is fresh? If they can't, you should take your business elsewhere.

Figuring Out What's Fresh

- The fish's eyes should be clear and bulge a little. Only a few fish, such as walleye, have naturally cloudy eyes.

- Whole fish and fillets should have firm and shiny flesh. Dull flesh may mean the fish is old. Fresh whole fish also should have bright red gills free from slime.

- If the flesh doesn't spring back when pressed, the fish isn't fresh. There should be no darkening around the edges of the fish or brown or yellowish discoloration.

- The fish should smell fresh and mild, not fishy or ammonia-like.

— by Paula Kurtzweil

Paula Kurtzweil is a member of FDA's public affairs staff.

Chapter 5

Safer Eggs:
Laying the Groundwork

The egg—long noted for its high quality protein and versatility in cooking—is getting a beating like no other.

At stake is its image as a safe and nutritious food.

In recent years, the egg has gained notoriety as a carrier of dangerous disease-causing *Salmonella* bacteria and as a food laden with artery-clogging cholesterol. Many of its best features—like ease of use, good taste, functionality, and low cost—have been lost in the stir.

But various groups, including the Food and Drug Administration and other government agencies, industry members, and nutrition educators, are fighting back. They are seeking to improve the safety of egg production and distribution through regulation and recommendations. They are educating people on the hazards of eating raw and undercooked eggs, urging them to adopt safe egg-handling practices and reminding them of the egg's importance in a healthful diet.

Cracking Down

Because eggs go through many channels and are handled in many ways before reaching someone's plate, FDA and the U.S. Department of Agriculture's Food Safety and Inspection Service (FSIS) announced in May 1998 that they would seek to identify "farm-to-table actions" to decrease the food safety risks associated with shell eggs. The agencies said they would consider regulations or guidance to cover egg

---

FDA Consumer, Sept./Oct. 1998; U.S. Food and Drug Administration.

handling on the farm, in transit, and at the retail level and asked for public comment on such topics as:

• federal quality assurance standards for egg production

• feasibility of large-scale use of an in-shell pasteurization process, a relatively new technology

• incentives to encourage egg refrigeration before transit

• the federal government's role in regulating restaurants and retail stores. Currently, federal agencies provide guidance, such as FDA's model *Food Code*, a reference for retail outlets on how to prepare food to prevent foodborne illness. FDA encourages states to adopt the *Food Code* as law.

In the May 19 advance notice of proposed rulemaking, FDA and FSIS announced that they would propose regulations "shortly" to improve the safety of eggs. The FSIS proposal would require eggs packed for consumer use to be refrigerated during distribution at a temperature not to exceed 45° F (7° C) and to include a label on packages that refrigeration is needed.

FDA's proposals would require:

• retail food stores and food service establishments to hold shell eggs at a refrigeration temperature of 45° F (7° C)

• safe handling instructions on the package labels of shell eggs that have not been treated to kill *Salmonella*. The instructions might say, for example, that raw eggs may contain harmful bacteria known to cause serious illness, especially in children, the elderly, and people with weakened immune systems. Consumers should be advised to keep eggs refrigerated and cook them thoroughly before eating.

Stopping the Outbreaks

While poultry, meat, fresh produce, and other raw foods also can be carriers of *Salmonella enteritidis* (SE), shell eggs lead the list. According to a study in the 1994 *Journal of Infectious Diseases*, 82 percent of SE outbreaks between 1985 and 1991 in which the vehicle for transmission was known were traced to contaminated shell eggs.

As many as 1 in 20,000 eggs, or about 2.7 million eggs annually in the United States, contains the bacteria, according to USDA.

Contamination occurs as the egg develops in the oviduct—the canal through which the egg travels—of an SE-infected chicken or from chicken fecal matter coming into contact with an egg.

FDA and FSIS' pending proposals and any other possible action they may take will help unify or supplement efforts already under way to prevent the spread of SE in eggs. For example, 38 states now require refrigeration of eggs at the retail level. And a number of states, including Ohio, California, Pennsylvania, and Maine and other Northeastern states, along with the United Egg Producers, an egg producers' cooperative, have established voluntary quality assurance programs for egg producers. Participants agree to follow certain practices, which may include:

- cleaning and disinfecting hen houses between flocks—adopting strict rodent control measures

- washing eggs properly

- refrigerating eggs between transport and storage

- putting in place biosecurity measures.

- monitoring mortality of chickens

- using SE-free chicks and pullets.

Also, the U.S. Animal Health Association, a professional association of veterinarians, has developed SE reduction guidelines for egg producers.

The Importance of Eggs

There are plenty of reasons to go to these lengths. A chief one is that eggs are one of the cheapest yet most nutritious foods around. For about 10 cents, an egg provides 6 grams of protein and substantial amounts of several important vitamins and minerals, such as vitamins A and B12, folate, thiamin, riboflavin, phosphorus, and zinc. The protein is of the highest quality, higher even than that of milk, meat and fish.

"Eggs are the gold standard of protein," says Liz Ward, a registered dietitian with the Harvard Vanguard Medical Association in Boston and spokeswoman for the American Dietetic Association.

Like meat, fish, milk, and other complete proteins, eggs provide all the essential amino acids needed to support life and growth.

Eggs also have several physical and chemical properties important in cooking and baking. Eggs thicken custards, puddings and sauces. They stabilize mayonnaise and salad dressings. They're often used to coat or glaze breads and cookies. They bind ingredients in foods like meatloaf and lasagna, clarify soups, prevent crystallization in boiled candies and frostings, and serve as leavening agents, helping foods like soufflés and sponge cakes to rise.

"There are a lot of things you can't make without eggs," says Betsy Crosby, a home economist with USDN's Agricultural Marketing Service.

Eggs also are easy to use. Because they can be cooked alone or, in many cases, with other foods relatively quickly, they are a convenient, nutritious food for people on the go and those unable to do much cooking. And, unlike other animal foods, they can keep in the refrigerator for three to five weeks.

Also, because eggs are soft and easy to chew, they are a good substitute for meat and other hard-to-chew protein-rich foods for anyone who has difficulty chewing.

However, because of an egg's cholesterol content—215 milligrams all contained in the yolk—the Dietary Guidelines for Americans recommends using egg yolks "in moderation." Egg whites contain no cholesterol (but all the protein) and can be used freely.

Pinpointing the Problem

State and federal investigators have traced *Salmonella enteritidis* outbreaks to various raw and undercooked egg-containing products, including Caesar salad, homemade Jamaican malt, French toast, lasagna, hollandaise sauce, and baked and sunnyside-up eggs. A major nationwide SE outbreak in 1994 involved ice cream, which, according to FDA's best determination, became contaminated during shipment of the ice cream mix in an improperly cleaned tanker previously used to haul unpasteurized liquid eggs. Also, the ice cream maker failed to repasteurize the ice cream mix after shipment.

Egg dishes made from "pooled" eggs, especially in institutional settings such as nursing homes, have been a frequent culprit. One contaminated raw egg can infect the whole lot when mixed together, for example, in making scrambled eggs.

SE is destroyed by cooking the egg or egg-containing dish to at least 145° F (63° C). In most of the SE outbreaks in the United States, the egg products were not cooked to the proper temperature.

Frequently, the eggs involved also were not held at a refrigeration temperature of 45° F (7° C) before cooking. Proper refrigeration can help prevent the growth of SE.

The cumulative effect of these errors often causes the outbreak.

In addition to government regulations, efforts under way to stop these errors and subsequent outbreaks include educating consumers, retail food handlers, and food service personnel about proper egg and other food handling.

Technological Advances

Modern technology also may aid in the effort. According to Marilyn Balmer, V.M.D., a consumer safety officer in FDA's Office of Plant and Dairy Foods and Beverages, FDA has reviewed processes for in-shell egg pasteurization, and one of several companies interested in offering it has test-marketed pasteurized in-shell eggs.

The marketability of such eggs is unknown because, home economist Crosby says, "This technology, if perfected, might be a tad expensive." But Charles Beard, D.V.M., Ph.D., vice president of research technology for the U.S. Poultry and Egg Association, points out that in-shell eggs are retailers' preferred product. "Shell eggs get more money [than liquid egg products]," he says.

Other technological possibilities include:

- ionizing radiation, also known as irradiation (see "Irradiation: A Safe Measure for Safer Food" in the May-June 1998 *FDA Consumer*), to reduce *Salmonella* in shell eggs. At press time, a food additive petition for such a use was under FDA review.

- reducing *Salmonella* in chickens by spraying newly hatched chickens with Preempt, a biotechnology product FDA approved last March that contains 29 bacteria. The bacteria, which the chicks ingest when they peck at their wet feathers, reduce *Salmonella* colonization in the chicks' intestines.

Technology may go a long way towards reducing *Salmonella enteritidis* in eggs, but Balmer says that, at present, "the problem is multifaceted. That's why the solution has to be a farm-to-table continuum."

Safe Egg Handling

To prevent infection with *Salmonella enteritidis*, follow these rules when buying, storing, preparing, serving, and eating eggs:

- Don't eat raw eggs. This includes so-called "health-food" beverages made with raw eggs, and foods traditionally made with raw eggs, such as Caesar salad, hollandaise sauce, homemade mayonnaise, ice cream, eggnog, and cookie dough, unless the dish was made with a pasteurized liquid egg product or pasteurized in-shell eggs. Egg mixtures made with an egg-milk base cooked to an internal temperature of 160° F (71° C) are safe, too. Use a thermometer to make sure the mixtures reach the correct temperature.

- Buy eggs only if sold in the grocer's refrigerated case. Open the carton and check that the eggs are clean and uncracked.

- Store eggs in their carton in the coldest part of the refrigerator, not in the door, and use within three to five weeks. The refrigerator should be set at 40° F (5° C) or slightly below.

- Keep hard-cooked eggs, including dyed Easter eggs, in the refrigerator, not at room temperature. Use within one week.

- Eggs should not be frozen in their shells. To freeze whole eggs, beat yolks and whites together. Egg whites also can be frozen by themselves. Use frozen eggs within one year.

- Wash hands, utensils, equipment, and work areas with warm, soapy water before and after contact with eggs and egg-rich foods.

- Don't leave cooked eggs out of the refrigerator for more than two hours. When baking or cooking, take out the eggs you need, and then return the carton to the refrigerator.

- Cook eggs until yolks are firm.

Additional information on safe egg and other food-handling practices is available from:

FDA

Office of Consumer Affairs
HFE-88
Rockville, MD 20857

FDA's Food Information Line
1-800-FDA-4010; (202) 205-4314 in the Washington, D.C. area
24 hours a day

FDA Website
www. cfsan.fda.gov/~mow/foodborn.html

USDA

Meat and Poultry Hotline
1-800-535-A555
(202) 720-3333 in the Washington, D.C., area
Recorded messages available 24 hours a day. Home economists and
registered dietitians available 10 a.m. to 4 p.m. Eastern time, Monday
through Friday.
www.fsis.usda.gov/OA/consedu.htm

Salmonella Threat

Salmonella is commonly found in the intestinal tracts of animals,
especially birds and reptiles. (See "The Fright of the Iguana" in the
November-December 1997 *FDA Consumer*.) In humans, *Salmonella*
infection can cause salmonellosis, an illness characterized by fever,
stomach cramps and diarrhea, which typically develop eight hours to
three days after eating a contaminated food or drink. The illness can
last as long as seven days, and severe cases may require hospitalization. In some people, it can cause death. A small number of illnesses
may develop into recurring joint pain and arthritis.

The degree to which a person becomes sick depends on his or her
health status and the number of bacteria ingested. The poorer the
health and the larger the number of bacteria, the greater the likelihood for serious illness. People who are most susceptible are children,
older Americans, and people with weakened immunity (for example,
people with AIDS or cancer).

Salmonella enteritidis is one of the major *Salmonella* strains show-
ing up in food. Between 1976 and 1994, the proportion of reported
Salmonella isolates that were this particular strain increased from 5
percent to 26 percent, according to the national Centers for Disease
Control and Prevention.

—by Paula Kurtzweil

Paula Kurtzweil is a member of FDA's public affairs staff.

Chapter 6

Critical Controls for Juice Safety

Fresh squeezed orange juice. Sparkling apple cider. All-vegetable cocktail. Americans quench their thirst with these and other fruit and vegetable juices, and the vast majority of those juices are not only healthy but safe. Very rarely, however, juice can turn dangerous.

Such was the 1996 case of a 16 month-old child in Colorado who died of heart damage and kidney failure after drinking contaminated apple juice. In another 1996 case involving contaminated apple juice, 3½-year-old Amanda Berman of Chicago was hospitalized for 24 days. In both cases, the apple juice was unpasteurized and the culprit was *E. coli* 0157: H7, the same microbe that claimed the lives of four children during a 1993 outbreak from undercooked hamburger.

This strain of *E. coli*, according to the national Centers for Disease Control and Prevention, is the most worrisome food-related threat to public health. Unlike other foodborne pathogens, *E. coli* 0157:H7 has no margin for error. It takes only a microscopic amount to cause serious illness or even death. In fact, CDC estimates that *E. coli* 0157:H7 bacteria are responsible for at least 20,000 cases of severe foodborne illness in the United States each year.

Because certain food poisoning outbreaks have been traced to fresh juices that were not pasteurized or otherwise processed to eliminate harmful bacteria, the Food and Drug Administration proposed in April measures to reduce the risk of illness from disease-causing microbes in unpasteurized fruit and vegetable juices.

FDA Consumer, Sept./Oct. 1998; U.S. Food and Drug Administration.

HACCP—A Tried and True Measure

Traditionally, industry and regulators have depended on spot-checks of manufacturing establishments and random sampling of final products to ensure safe foods. While these inspections provide a general picture of circumstances at the time, little is known about conditions before and after the inspections, as well as beyond the facility, which can all have a bearing on the safety of the finished product.

A 1997 study by FDA's Center for Food Safety and Applied Nutrition found that while contamination of juice products most likely occurs during the growing and harvesting of the raw product, it may occur at any point between the orchard and the table. Therefore, FDA's proposed regulations will require juice processors to implement a Hazard Analysis and Critical Control Point (HACCP) plan that addresses all points of production.

HACCP is a science-based system designed to prevent, reduce or eliminate hazards in food products through appropriate controls during production and processing. Key components of the system include:

- identifying potential problems that could cause food to be unsafe to eat

- establishing and monitoring targeted control points to minimize such problems

- documenting the results

In addition to a number of U.S. food companies already using individually tailored HACCP systems in their manufacturing processes, systems are also in place in Canada and in other countries.

"Since 1973, there have been no reported cases of botulism in foods processed under FDA's low-acid canned foods regulations, which is based on the HACCP principle," says Shellee Davis, a consumer safety officer with FDA's Office of Plant and Dairy Foods and Beverages. "We think an adequate HACCP program is an effective way to ensure that juices are safe as well."

Warning Label Required

In addition to HACCP, a warning is now required on unpasteurized juices. This warning, part of the April proposal, was published as a final rule on July 8.

The warning label must be visible on the information panel or on the principal display panel of the container's label and must read: "WARNING: This product has not been pasteurized and, therefore may contain harmful bacteria that can cause serious illness in children, the elderly, and persons with weakened immune systems." For apple juice or apple cider, the warning statement is required beginning Sept. 8. For all other unpasteurized juices, the effective date is Nov. 5, 1999.

"The new labeling is only intended to be an interim measure [because] we have proposed a 3-year phase-in period for processors to implement their HACCP programs," says LeeAnn Jackson, Ph.D., a science policy analyst with the Center for Food Safety and Applied Nutrition's executive operations staff. "Large manufacturers will be given one year while small and very small businesses will be given two and three years, respectively," she added.

What Can Consumers Do?

FDA urges high-risk individuals—children, the elderly, and those with weakened immune systems—to drink only pasteurized juices. And while manufacturers were asked before the date in the regulation to voluntarily place warning statements on the labels of juices that haven't been pasteurized, the agency advises people to be aware that a product without a warning label at this time might still be unpasteurized. A good rule of thumb for high-risk individuals, says FDA, is if you cannot determine whether a product has been pasteurized, the best choice is to not use the product. Another choice is to bring the juice to a boil to kill any possible harmful bacteria.

The agency also advises consumers to be aware of the following symptoms commonly associated with food poisoning: diarrhea, abdominal pain, cramping, vomiting, fever, and headache. If you have any of these symptoms, you should contact your physician immediately.

The Future of HACCP

New challenges arising from the growing size of the food industry and the diversity of products and processes have prompted FDA to consider requiring HACCP regulations as a standard throughout much of the remaining U.S. food supply. If adopted, the regulations would cover both domestic and imported foods.

"Any process that helps eliminate contamination in our food and beverages is a positive sign," says Adam Berman, who also said his daughter Amanda, now 5, is recovering well from her illness. "I'd like to think that there is no way we would forego or compromise any precautions necessary to ensure safe foods."

—by Carol Lewis

Carol Lewis is a staff writer for *FDA Consumer*.

To Pasteurize or Not to Pasteurize

FDA is aware of the significant benefits of pasteurizing juice, as well as the reasons some processors choose not to do so. Pasteurization is the process of heat-treating liquid or semi-liquid foods to a temperature for a designated period sufficient to destroy certain disease or food-spoilage bacteria. In the United States, 98 percent of all fruit and vegetable juices are pasteurized. Still, some processors believe that pasteurization alters the flavor of a product and degrades its nutritional value.

The Center for Food Safety and Applied Nutrition found in its preliminary study that unpasteurized juices accounted for 76 percent of contamination cases reported between 1993 and 1996. In addition, the study concluded that illnesses associated with unpasteurized juices tended to be more severe than those associated with pasteurized products. Therefore, FDA believes that pasteurization, or a comparable process that would eliminate or reduce the level of harmful pathogens that can cause food-borne illness, appears to offer an effective way to control the significant hazards that have become a problem with juice.

—C. L.

Not All Juices Are Created Equal

If you don't want to concentrate all your strength on choosing a juice, the Information below will help make the choice easier:

100% Pure or 100% Juice: Guarantees only 100 percent fruit juice, complete with all its nutrients. If it's not there, it's not all juice.

Fresh Squeezed Juice: Squeezed from fresh fruit. It is not pasteurized and is usually located in the produce or dairy section of the grocery store.

"Cocktail," "Punch," "Drink," "Beverage": Terms that signify diluted juice containing less than 100 percent juice, often with added sweeteners.

From Concentrate: Water is removed from whole juice to make concentrate; then water is added back to reconstitute to 100 percent juice or to diluted juice such as lemonade.

Not From Concentrate: Juice that has never been concentrated.

Fresh Frozen: Freshly squeezed, and packaged and frozen without pasteurization or further processing. It is usually sold in plastic bottles in the frozen food section of the grocery store and is ready to drink after thawing.

Juice on Unrefrigerated Shelves: Shelf-stable product usually found with canned and bottled juices on unrefrigerated shelves of your store. It is pasteurized juice, or diluted juice, often from concentrate, packaged in sterilized containers.

Canned Juice: Heated and sealed in cans to provide extended shelf life of more than one year.

Chapter 7

Pesticides in Foods

Pesticide residues on infant foods and adult foods that infants and children eat are almost always well below tolerances (the highest levels legally allowed) set by the Environmental Protection Agency. This was the conclusion of a recent Food and Drug Administration report based on the agency's monitoring of these types of foods over the last seven years.

The FDA report, "Monitoring of Pesticide Residues in Infant Foods and Adult Foods Eaten by Infants and Children," was published in May-June 1993 issue of the *Journal of the Association of Official Analytical Chemists International.*

The authors, consumer safety officer Norma Yess and chemists Ellis Gunderson and Ronald Roy of the Center for Food Safety and Applied Nutrition, based their findings on food samples from the three approaches FDA uses to monitor pesticides: Regulatory, incidence and level, and Total Diet Study.

Through the regulatory approach, FDA checks foods close to the point of production for levels of residues and, if they are violative, considers enforcement action. Incidence and level is a study approach that analyzes selected samples of certain foods. Total Diet Study is an approach that uses data from supermarket shopping.

Of more than 10,000 food samples reported from regulatory monitoring, fewer than 50 were violative. No residues over EPA and FDA action levels were found in samples from the incidence and level

---

FDA Consumer 1993; Food and Drug Administration.

studies. In the Total Diet Study, no residues were found in infant formulas, and no residues over FDA or EPA allowed levels were found.

Shared Responsibility

The responsibility for ensuring that residues of pesticides in foods are not present at levels that will pose a danger to health is shared by FDA, EPA, and the Food Safety and Inspection Service of the U.S. Department of Agriculture. Pesticides of concern include insecticides, fungicides, herbicides, and other agricultural chemicals.

EPA reviews the scientific data on all pesticide products before they can be registered (or licensed) for use. If a product is intended for use on food crops, EPA also establishes a tolerance.

FDA is responsible for enforcing these tolerances on all foods except meat, poultry, and certain egg products, which are monitored by USDA. In addition, FDA works with EPA to set "action levels"—enforcement guidelines for residues of pesticides, such as DDT, that may remain in the environment after their use is discontinued. The guidelines are set at levels the protect public health.

Regulatory Monitoring

In its regulatory monitoring to enforce EPA-set tolerances, FDA checks foods for pesticide residues as close to production of the commodity as possible—at distributors, at food processors, or, if imported, at entry into the country. If illegal residues are found in domestic samples, FDA can take regulatory action, such as seizure or injunction. For imports, FDA can stop shipments at ports of entry.

The FDA report used data from FDA regulatory monitoring between 1985 and 1991. The authors chose eight foods that infants and children eat in relatively large quantities—apples, bananas, oranges and pears; apple, grape and orange juice; and milk. FDA found 50 violative samples, representing only 0.3 percent of domestic products and 0.6 percent of imports reported under the regulatory monitoring approach.

All food samples in regulatory monitoring are analyzed unwashed and unpeeled—even bananas. Yess explains that because food processors, and most consumers, wash or peel produce before eating or using it in food products, many of the violative samples reported in the FDA study showed higher residues that the actual amount people are exposed to. Studies have shown that residues of many pesticides can be washed off fresh produce, a good practice for anyone fixing a salad or snacking on grapes (refer to end of chapter).

Of the 50 violative samples, nearly all were pesticide residues for which there were no tolerances of EPA "approval for use" on the specific food sampled. Since pesticides are registered for specific crops, residues on crops for which the pesticide has not been registered are illegal.

A few samples had residues higher than EPA tolerances or FDA action levels in effect at the time; a number of tolerances were revised between 1985 and 1991. The revisions for daminozide (Alar), for example, reflect that it has not been used in agriculture since 1989.

Some domestic milk samples showed small amounts of chlorinated pesticide residues. The registration for food use for these compounds expired more than 20 years ago, but because they persist in the environment, residues are still found at low levels.

Incidence and Level Studies

When FDA wants to know more about specific pesticides, commodities, or pesticide-commodity combinations, the agency supplements its regulatory monitoring by analyzing selected samples of certain foods in incidence and level monitoring.

For the pesticide residue report, the authors used the results of two studies. One study targeted five specific commodity-pesticide combinations for infant foods and foods commonly eaten by infants and children. The analyses for this study were directed by FDA and completed in 1990, analyzed whole pasteurized milk samples through an FDA-supported contract.

Both studies included results of analyses of several pesticides and pesticide-commodity combinations that was the focus of public attention within the last five years. No residues over EPA tolerances of FDA action levels were found in samples from either of the two studies.

The first study involved five tasks. In the first, about 900 samples of commercially prepared infant foods and formulas were collected and analyzed for residues of the following pesticides:

- benomyl-thiabendazole (fungicides)

- daminozide (sprayed on apple trees to prevent premature drop, no longer used by growers)

- ethylenethiourea (ETU, a breakdown product of a fungicide)

- aldicarb (an insecticide, acaricide against snails, and nematocide against worms)

- the organochlorine group of pesticides, including those no longer used in foods).

The other four tasks were analyses of adult foods eaten by infants and children:

- apples, bananas, oranges, and pears for benomyl-thiabendazole

- apple and grape juices, applesauce, and canned pear for daminozide

- grape juice for ETU

- bananas, oranges, and orange juice for aldicarb.

These quarters of the samples collected for all tasks were from large retail grocery stores in six states—Massachusetts, Illinois, Michigan, Wisconsin, Minnesota, and Washington. The remaining samples were collected in the Gulfport, Miss., area (the home of USDA's National Monitoring and Residues Analysis Laboratory, where the FDA-directed study was done). The prepared infant foods and formula samples were selected mostly from the major manufacturers.

The second study showed the results of sampling for residues of the organochlorine group of pesticides in whole pasteurized milk. Organochlorine pesticide residues—mostly DDT, DDE and dieldrin—were found in 398 of the 806 milk samples, but all were well below EPA tolerances or FDA action levels.

Samples for the milk study came from monthly collections at 63 sampling stations that are a part of EPA's Environmental Radiation Ambient Monitoring Systems, located in large metropolitan areas throughout the United States. At each sampling station, milk from selected sources was combined to represent the milk routinely consumed in that area. Portions of the milk were sent to an FDA contract laboratory for analysis.

Total Diet Study

For its report, FDA also used data from the Total Diet Study, which is used to monitor a number of nutritional concerns, including pesticides. As part of the Total Diet Study, FDA staffers shop in supermarket or grocery stores four times a year, once in each of four geographical regions of the country. Shopping in three cities from each region, they buy the same 234 foods (including meat), selected from nationwide dietary survey data to typify the American diet. The purchased foods are called "market baskets."

Foods from the market baskets are then prepared as a consumer would prepare them. For example, beef and vegetable stew is made from the collected ingredients, using a standard recipe. The prepared foods are analyzed for pesticide residues, and the results, together with USDA consumption studies, are used to estimate the dietary intakes of pesticide residues for eight age-sex groups ranging from infants to senior citizens.

For their report, the FDA researchers included results from 27 market baskets collected and analyzed between 1985 and 1991. Included were 33 different infant foods (both strained and junior), 10 adult foods eaten by infants and children, and four types of milk. The infant foods included cereals, combination meat and poultry dinners, vegetables, desserts, fruits and fruit juices, and infant formulas. The adult foods included apples, oranges, pears, and bananas; apple, grape and orange juices; applesauce; grape jelly; and peanut butter. Milks were chocolate, evaporated, low-fat (2percent), and whole.

No residues were found in the infant formulas, and no residues over EPA tolerances or FDA action levels were found in any of the Total Diet Study foods. Low levels of malathion were found in some cereals because malathion is widely used both before and after harvest on grains. Low levels of thiabendazole, a post-harvest fungicide used on many fruits, were found on some of the fruits and fruit products.

The low levels of pesticide residues found in the Total Diet Study and incidence-level monitoring samples show how processing foods or otherwise preparing them for consumption at the table can reduce residue levels. Washing at home removes much of the residues. But commercial food processing steps, such as peeling and blanching, can further reduce residues. For example, the highest finding of thiabendazole in raw apples was 2 parts per million (EPA tolerance is 10ppm), 0.08 in apple juice, and 0.06 in applesauce. Also, agricultural specialists from major infant food manufacturers work with their contract growers to minimize pesticide applications and to ensure that only those pesticides specified in the contract are applied. Therefore, when pesticide residues are found on infant foods, they are usually well below EPA tolerances.

Wash Before Eating

Washing fresh produce before eating is a healthful habit. You can reduce and often eliminate residues if they are present on fresh fruits and vegetables by following these simple tips:

- Wash produce with large amounts of cold or warm tap water, and scrub with a brush when appropriate; do not use soap.

- Throw away the outer leaves of leafy vegetables such as lettuce and cabbage.

- Trim the fat from meat, and fat and skin from poultry and fish. Residues of some pesticides concentrate in animal fat.

Supermarkets, as a rule, don't wash produce before putting it out, but many stores mist it while it is on display. Misting keeps the produce from drying, but surface residues drain off also, in much the same way as from a light was under the kitchen faucet.

A 1990 report in the EPA Journal by three chemists from the agency, Joel Garbus, Susan Hummel, and Stephanie Willet, summarized four studies of fresh tomatoes treated with a fungicide, which were tested a harvest, at the packing house, and at point of sale to the consumer. The studies showed that more than 99 percent of the residues were washed off at the packing house by the food processor.

A 1989 study reported by Edgar Elkins in the *Journal of the Association of Official Analytical Chemists* showed the effects of peeling, blanching and processing on a number of fruits and vegetables. For example, in the case of benomyl, 83 percent of the residues found on fresh apples were removed during processing into applesauce, 98 percent of residues from oranges processed to juice were removed, and 86 percent of residues from fresh tomatoes processed to juice were removed. Another study in 1991 by Gary Eilrich, reported in an American Chemical Society Symposium, showed similar results.

Chapter 8

Should "Pre-Washed" Salad Greens Be Washed Again?

More than a year's worth of scary television and newspaper reports about high bacterial counts in pre-cut, pre-packaged salad greens have left consumers wondering. Is the convenience of read-to-serve, fresh lettuce in a bag worth the risk of contracting a deadly foodborne illness like *E. coli* infection? The question goes to the heart of how best to stay healthy, since the case of tossing pre-mixed salad fixings into a bowl has been attracting people who might not otherwise be eating all the greens that health experts now say, can ward off diseases such as certain types of cancer.

The salad scare originally began with an article in a major newspaper. Staff there purchased different types of pre-cut vegetables, including several pre-packaged salads, and sent them to a lab to be tested for bacteria. The result: high bacterial levels were indeed found in a number of products.

The stations across the country soon picked up the story, doing tests of their own and getting the same results. "For some—this so called convenient food may not be worth the trouble," said one investigator. Another report contained the statement, "You're probably better off eating raw ground beef than you are eating this produce."

But the lab results obtained first by the newspaper and then by other media were misinterpreted. That's because what were found were high levels of innocuous bacteria belonging to the coliform group—distant and altogether harmless relatives of deadly strains of *E. coli*. It's not surprising. Nothing grown in the ground, including vegetables, can be completely sterile.

"High-quality produce will normally contain at least 10,000 harmless microorganisms per gram—and that number can range up to 10 million," says Larry Beuchat, PhD, of the Center for Food Safety and Quality Enhancement at the University of Georgia. "That may sound startling to some people, but it's a fact. High bacterial counts aren't alarming by themselves—it's the type of bacteria, not the numbers, that are of most concern."

In fact, coliforms and other bacteria keep produce safe by competing with more dangerous bacteria for nutrients. Not only does that cut down on the growth rate of harmful "bugs," but it also helps to ensure that produce will spoil and then be thrown out before it could sicken someone. That's because when harmless bacteria multiply, they form a slime on lettuce leaves and turn them brown.

"It's like a built-in alert system," says Dr. Beuchat. "The product will become inedible before enough illness-causing microorganisms could grow."

So Can a Salad Go Straight From Bag to Bowl?

The fact that lab results were misinterpreted doesn't mean all premixed salad greens that look good enough to eat can be emptied into your bowl without washing. Consider that most supermarkets carry two kinds of pre-cut lettuce: the packaged kind, which comes in a sealed plastic bag, and bulk lettuce (also known as spring or mesclun mix), which is usually displayed in bins where shoppers use tongs to select their own assortment of leaves.

Bulk lettuce should always be washed—even if it looks ready to eat and even if the box in which it's displayed says "washed." Any produce that's sold out in the open, where people can touch it or sneeze on it, is subject to contamination by harmful bacteria in the store— or could have picked them up along the way as it was packed and shipped from the fields. and the consequences of eating it without first giving it two or three careful rinses could be dire. Pretty looking, but unclean bulk lettuce, that was packed on a small lettuce farm in California and distributed to restaurants and retail stores in Connecticut, Illinois, and New York led to out breaks of *E. coli* infection in 1996 that caused at least 70 illnesses—some severe enough to send people to the hospital.

As far as bagged salads go, however, "there's been no evidence of a problem, ever, with pre-packaged lettuce—the sealed, washed, ready-to-eat type," says Jeff Farrar, DVM, MPH, a scientist at the California Department of Public Health Government officials at both the U.S. Department of Agriculture and the Centers for Disease Control and Prevention concur.

The words to look for on a plastic package of greens to make sure it has been washed thoroughly enough so that you don't have to wash it again: "washed" and "ready to eat." large manufacturers, including Dole, Ready-Pac, and Fresh Express, use this type of wording. They also use a state-of-the-art cleansing process that kills bacteria better than you could at home.

But don't automatically assume that every salad that comes in a sealed plastic bag has been pre-washed. One bag we came across, for example, boasted that the lettuce inside was fresh and sweet—but said nothing about the company's washing process. Words like "fresh," "natural," "organic," and "premium," while they may sound appealing, don't guarantee cleanliness. In such cases, where it's not clear whether the greens are ready to eat, you should definitely take the extra step of washing them.

Also make sure to follow the "Use By" date on the package, even if it carries the "washed" and "ready to eat" terms. Lettuce that has lingered too long in the store or at home could have deteriorated in quality no matter how well it was washed in the beginning.

Chapter 9

Possible Danger in Public Drinking Water

It's a warning we hope never to see in our kitchens, but recent research from the Johns Hopkins School of Public Health suggests that you might want to be a bit wary of public drinking water supplies because *Cryptosporidium parvum*, a water-borne parasite that can cause serious illness, may be lurking in it. InteliHealth spoke with Thaddeus K. Graczyk, Ph.D., an assistant scientist in the Department of Molecular Microbiology and Immunology at the Johns Hopkins School of Public Health, about this potential contaminant of our drinking water.

What Is Cryptosporidium and How Serious Is Its Threat?

Cryptosporidium is a waterborne zoonotic parasite that comprises eight species, only one of which, *C. parvum*, is infectious to humans. Up to 60 percent of us have been exposed to *C. parvum*, and normally the illness it causes, called cryptosporidiosis, involves diarrhoeal disease, which is self-limiting in healthy, immunocompetent individuals. However, people with impaired immune systems, such as those who are HIV-seropositive, are at significant risk of dying from it, and young children may also be seriously affected.

How Does C. parvum *Get Into the Water Supply?*

The trouble often starts with cows. If rain runoff washes bovine feces containing the parasitic spores of *C. parvum* into water supplies, then the microscopic spores can often slip through water treatment facilities like fine sand through a screen. Also, manure spread on fields can contaminate surface water when washed off with rains. Birds, particularly waterfowl, can also spread the spores, so that autumn may be a particularly vulnerable period for watersheds: when migratory waterfowl stop over in a watershed area, they can act as a "mechanical vector," excreting *C. parvum* into the reservoirs that hold our drinking water. Thus, a flock of visiting Canada geese, while helping meet wildlife conservation goals, can also have disease implications for humans.

What Can This Microbe Do to Humans?

Cryptosporidiosis is characterized by acute watery diarrhea, fever, abdominal pain, and fatigue. In immunocompromised people, watery diarrhea can be chronic and can significantly contribute to death.

Are the Initial Symptoms Serious Enough So That People Seek Help Before It's Too Late? And Can Most Doctors Readily Diagnose it? Are There Any Treatments For It?

Clinical symptoms should alert the patient to seek professional help. Infection can be diagnosed by laboratory findings of Cryptosporidium oocysts in the fecal specimen. There is, however, no effective pharmacological treatment for Cryptosporidium infection.

Have There Ever Been Any Large Outbreaks of Cryptosporidiosis?

An outbreak occurred in Milwaukee in 1993 that sickened 400,000 people when that city's water purification system failed to detect the pathogen. About 100 immunocompromised persons died as a result of the Milwaukee outbreak.

Are Water Treatment Facilities Getting Better at Detecting This Contamination and Stopping It?

Water treatment facilities routinely test for *C. parvum* by using something called an "immunofluorescent antibody assay" (IFA), but this test often yields false positives because it has trouble distinguishing among the eight species of Cryptosporidium. This of course alarms the public with erroneous reports of contaminated water, so it's important to distinguish between infectious and noninfectious species of Cryptosporidium. Here at the School of Public Health, we have tested a new method for identifying *C. parvum*, called "enzyme immunoassay" or EIA, and found it to be more accurate.

When Will That Test Be Deployed at Water Treatment Facilities?

EIA was designed to test fecal specimens for Cryptosporidium oocysts, so it's difficult to say when it will be deployed at water treatment facilities.

Once a City's Water Department Detects C. parvum, Can They Then Remove the Bug from the Water Supply?

When Cryptosporidium is detected, the water treatment procedures at the water treatment facility can be altered in order to remove and/or inactivate Cryptosporidium oocysts.

Can People do Anything at Home to Guarantee That Their Water Is Free of C. parvum?

Boiling drinking water for a full minute kills this pathogen. Or, buy bottled drinking water.

But Aren't Some Bottled "Spring" Waters Just Tap Water That's Been Bottled in Some Other Region of the Country and Then Shipped Out?

Although most bottled water is underground water, some brands labeled as "spring" water are surface water. One must call the manufacturer to be certain.

What about Some of the Home Filtration Systems for Water—Do Any of Them Catch Cryptosporidium?

Yes, some commercially available home filtration systems can. The label on the purchased filter should indicate that that particular device is capable of removing Cryptosporidium oocysts from the water.

With Global Warming, We are Beginning to See Many More Violent Thunderstorms and "Gullywashers," Which Dump an Inch or Two of Water on an Area in Just a Few Minutes. Are These Extreme Weather Events Affecting our Water Supply?

Yes, the flooding that accompanies extreme weather events can increase the chances of waterborne contamination with Cryptosporidium.

Chapter 10

Don't Get Bitten by the Travel Bug: Eat Safely Overseas

You've carefully planned and eagerly awaited this vacation for months. The last thing you want is to spend precious vacation time trapped in a bathroom because of diarrhea, nausea and cramps. Unfortunately this scenario is all too common; traveler's diarrhea strikes millions of Americans who go abroad each year.

Traveler's diarrhea is one of the most common types of foodborne illness suffered by Americans visiting other countries. It is caused by consuming food or water contaminated with human waste, which can carry harmful bacteria, viruses or parasites.

The condition is not generally life threatening, but it is debilitating. Though it typically lasts three to four days—just long enough to ruin a long-awaited trip abroad—the severity and duration of the illness depends on the type of toxin and the amount ingested. A bout of traveler's diarrhea can be over in 24 hours, or it can lay you up for a week or more.

Does Your Destination Spell Trouble?

Whether you'll be at risk on your vacation this summer depends on where you're going. Because western countries have strict regulations regarding sanitation and hygiene, traveler's diarrhea is uncommon in places like Canada, Northern Europe, New Zealand and Australia. On the other hand, in some developing countries in Latin

---

America, Africa, Asia and the Middle East, sanitation is questionable, making these destinations high-risk. In some places, as many as one of every two American visitors suffers the consequences of traveler's diarrhea.

Yet even in exotic locales, illness can be avoided by being careful about what you eat and drink. According to the Centers for Disease Control and Prevention (CDC) in Atlanta, the best advice is to stay away from raw or undercooked meat or seafood, as well as all raw produce, such as fruits, vegetables and salads, and of course, tap water.

"For the amount of time most people spend abroad, it's not going to be detrimental to their health if they don't eat fresh fruits and vegetables," says Robert Quick, M.D., an epidemiologist with the foodborne and diarrheal diseases branch at CDC.

If you want to sample native fresh fruits, buy a thick-skinned variety with the skin still on. Then peel it yourself. (Contaminated water could be clinging to the peel.)

Don't Drink the Water!

Water is a potential problem, even in some industrialized countries. A safe bet is to drink only commercially bottled, carbonated beverages (carbonation lowers acidity and kills some organisms), beer, wine or steaming hot coffee or tea. Avoid tap water altogether, even for brushing your teeth. And don't use ice. If you must use tap water, boil it first.

It's best to drink directly from a bottle or can you've opened yourself and to use a straw you've unwrapped. Wipe the top of the can or bottle before you open it to get rid of any contaminants that may be lurking on the outside. If you must drink from a glass, pour it yourself and be sure the glass is clean and dry.

Beware of Dairy

Even in developed countries, you're at risk for foodborne illness other than traveler's diarrhea. There have been a number of cases in the last few years of Americans in Europe getting sick from eating cheeses made from raw, unpasteurized milk. These cheeses can harbor the harmful bacteria *Listeria monocytogenes* or *Salmonella paratyphi*. Eating unpasteurized cheese that has not been aged at least six months is most risky for pregnant women, small children, the elderly and those with weakened immune systems.

Cheeses in Europe do not have to be labeled as unpasteurized. The best way to minimize your risk of getting sick overseas is to forgo any fresh, soft unripened cheese, such as Brie, Camembert, marscarpone and cottage cheese. Instead, opt for well-aged varieties like Cheddar, Parmesan, Asiago or Romano.

Common Sense Precautions

Be sure hot foods are hot and cold foods are cold, and that restaurants are scrupulously clean and neat. When dining out, look for reputable establishments like hotels or "fine dining" restaurants. Avoid places with dirty tabletops, utensils or plates. Also beware of waitstaff and cooks wearing soiled clothing. Check out the hands of foodservice workers-dirty fingernails are not a good sign. And beware of eating al fresco. "We recommend travelers don't eat food from street vendors in developing countries," notes Quick. "These people generally don't have access to running water. It's also very difficult to keep food heated properly."

"Our overall advice is boil it, cook it, peel it or forget it," says Quick, "aside from that, use common sense."

—by Diane Welland

Part Two

Common Foodborne Pathogens

Chapter 11

Onset, Duration, and Symptoms of Foodborne Illness

This chapter includes seven tables describing the approximate onset time to symptoms, the predominant symptoms, and associated organisms or toxins for various common foodborne illnesses. The tables, beginning on the next page, show information for:

- upper gastrointestinal tract symptoms (nausea, vomiting) occur first or predominate.

- sore throat and respiratory symptoms occur.

- lower gastrointestinal tract symptoms (abdominal cramps, diarrhea) occur first or predominate

- neurological symptoms (visual disturbances, vertigo, tingling, paralysis) occur.

- allergic symptoms (facial flushing, itching) cccur.

- generalized infection symptoms (fever, chills, malaise, prostration, aches, swollen lymph nodes) occur.

- gastrointestinal and/or neurologic symptoms—(shellfish toxins)

Foodborne Pathogenic Microorganisms and Natural Toxins Handbook, January 1992, U.S. Food & Drug Administration, Center for Food Safety & Applied Nutrition.

Table 11.1. Upper Gastrointestinal Tract Symptoms (Nausea, Vomiting) Occur First or Predominate.

Approximate onset time to symptoms	Predominant symptoms	Associated organism or toxin
Less than 1 hour	Nausea, vomiting, unusual taste, burning of mouth.	Metallic salts
1-2 hours	Nausea, vomiting, cyanosis, headache, dizziness, dyspnea, trembling, weakness, loss of consciousness.	Nitrites
1-6 hours mean 2-4 hours	Nausea, vomiting, retching, diarrhea, abdominal pain, prostration.	*Staphylococcus aureus* and its enterotoxins
8-16 hours (2-4 hours emesis possible)	Vomiting, abdominal cramps, diarrhea, nausea.	*Bacillus cereus*
6-24 hours	Nausea, vomiting, diarrhea, thirst, dilation of pupils, collapse, coma.	Amanita species mushrooms

Table 11.2. Sore Throat and Respiratory Symptoms Occur.

Approximate onset time to symptoms	Predominant symptoms	Associated organism or toxin
12-72 hours	Sore throat, fever, nausea vomiting, rhinorrhea, sometimes a rash.	*Streptococcus pyogenes*
2-5 days	Inflamed throat and nose, spreading grayish exudate, fever, chills, sore throat, malaise, difficulty in swallowing, edema of cervical lymph node.	*Corynebacterium diphtheriae*

Table 11.3. Lower Gastrointestinal Tract Symptoms (Abdominal Cramps, Diarrhea) Occur First or Predominate

Approximate onset time to symptoms	Predominant symptoms	Associated organism or toxin
2-36 hours, mean 6-12 hours	Abdominal cramps, diarrhea, putrefactive diarrhea associated with *C. perfringens*, sometimes nausea and vomiting.	*Clostridium perfringens, Bacillus cereus, Streptococcus faecalis, S. faecium*
12-74 hours, mean 18-36 hours	Abdominal cramps, diarrhea, vomiting, fever, chills, malaise, nausea, headache, possible. Sometimes bloody or mucoid diarrhea, cutaneous lesions associated with V. vulnificus. Yersinia enterocolitica mimics flu and acute appendicitis.	*Salmonella* species (including *S. arizonae, Shigella,* entero-pathogenic *Escherichia coli,* other *Enterobacteriacae, Vibrio parahaemolyticus, Yersinia enterocolitica, Pseudomonas aeruginosa*(?), *Aeromonas hydrophila, Plesiomonas shigelloides, Campylobacter jejuni, Vibrio cholerae* (O1 and non-O1), *V. vulnificus, V. fluvialis*
3-5 days	Diarrhea, fever, vomiting abdominal pain, respiratory symptoms.	Enteric viruses
1-6 weeks	Mucoid diarrhea (fatty stools) abdominal pain, weight loss.	*Giardia lamblia*
1 to several weeks	Abdominal pain, diarrhea, constipation, headache, drowsiness, ulcers, variable —often asymptomatic.	*Entamoeba histolytica*
3-6 months	Nervousness, insomnia, hunger pains, anorexia, weight loss, abdominal pain, sometimes gastroenteritis.	*Taenia saginata, T. solium*

83

Table 11.4. Neurological Symptoms (Visual Disturbances, Vertigo, Tingling, Paralysis) Occur.

Approximate onset time to symptoms	Predominant symptoms	Associated organism or toxin
Less than 1 hour	* See Gastrointestinal and/ or Neurologic Symptoms (Shellfish Toxins)	Shellfish toxin
	Gastroenteritis, nervousness, blurred vision, chest pain, cyanosis, twitching, convulsions.	Organic phosphate
	Excessive salivation, perspiration, gastroenteritis, irregular pulse, pupils constricted, asthmatic breathing.	Muscaria-type mushrooms
	Tingling and numbness, dizziness, pallor, gastrohemmorrhage, and desquamation of skin, fixed eyes, loss of reflexes, twitching, paralysis.	Tetradon (tetrodotoxin) toxins
1-6 hours	Tingling and numbness, gastroenteritis, dizziness, dry mouth, muscular aches, dilated pupils, blurred vision, paralysis.	Ciguatera toxin
	Nausea, vomiting, tingling, dizziness, weakness, anorexia, weight loss, confusion.	Chlorinated hydrocarbons
2 hours to 6 days, usually 12-36 hours	Vertigo, double or blurred vision, loss of reflex to light, difficulty in swallowing, speaking, and breathing, dry mouth, weakness, respiratory paralysis.	*Clostridium botulinum* and its neurotoxins
More than 72 hours	Numbness, weakness of legs, spastic paralysis, impairment of vision, blindness, coma.	Organic mercury
	Gastroenteritis, leg pain, ungainly high-stepping gait, foot and wrist drop.	Triorthocresyl phosphate

Table 11.5. Allergic Symptoms (Facial Flushing, Itching) Occur.

Approximate onset time to symptoms	Predominant symptoms	Associated organism or toxin
Less than 1 hour	Headache, dizziness, nausea, vomiting, peppery taste, burning of throat, facial swelling and flushing, stomach pain, itching of skin.	Histamine (scombroid)
	Numbness around mouth, tingling sensation, flushing, dizziness, headache, nausea.	Monosodium glutamate
	Flushing, sensation of warmth, itching, abdominal pain, puffing of face and knees.	Nicotinic acid

Table 11.6. Generalized Infection Symptoms (Fever, Chills, Malaise, Prostration, Aches, Swollen Lymph Nodes) Occur.

Approximate onset time to symptoms	Predominant symptoms	Associated organism or toxin
4-28 days, mean 9 days	Gastroenteritis, fever, edema about eyes, perspiration, muscular pain, chills, prostration, labored breathing.	*Trichinella spiralis*
7-28 days, mean 14 days	Malaise, headache, fever, cough, nausea, vomiting, constipation, abdominal pain, chills, rose spots, bloody stools.	*Salmonella typhi*
10-13 days	Fever, headache, myalgia, rash.	*Toxoplasma gondii*
10-50 days, mean 25-30 days	Fever, malaise, lassitude, anorexia, nausea, abdominal pain, jaundice.	Etiological agent not yet isolated— probably viral
Varying periods (depends on specific illness)	Fever, chills, head- or joint ache, prostration, malaise, swollen lymph nodes, and other specific symptoms of disease in question.	*Bacillus anthracis, Brucella melitensis, B. abortus, B. suis, Coxiella burnetii, Francisella tularensis, Listeria monocytogenes, Mycobacterium tuberculosis, Mycobacterium* species, *Pasteurella multocida, Streptobacillus moniliformis, Campylobacter jejuni, Leptospira* species.

Table 11.7. Gastrointestinal and/or Neurologic Symptoms—(Shellfish Toxins)

Approximate onset time to symptoms	Predominant symptoms	Associated organism or toxin
0.5 to 2 hours	Tingling, burning, numbness, drowsiness, incoherent speech, respiratory paralysis	Paralytic Shellfish Poisoning (PSP) (saxitoxins)
2-5 min to 3-4 hours	Reversal of hot and cold sensation, tingling; numbness of lips, tongue and throat; muscle aches, dizziness, diarrhea, vomiting	Neurotoxic Shellfish Poisoning (NSP) (brevetoxins)
30 min to 2-3 hours	Nausea, vomiting, diarrhea, abdominal pain, chills, fever	Diarrheic Shellfish Poisoning (DSP) (dinophysis toxin, okadaic acid, pectenotoxin, yessotoxin)
24 hours (gastrointestinal) to 48 hours (neurologic)	Vomiting, diarrhea, abdominal pain, confusion, memory loss, disorientation, seizure, coma	Amnesic Shellfish Poisoning (ASP) (domoic acid)

Chapter 12

Salmonella

Name of the Organism

Salmonella spp. Salmonella is a rod-shaped, motile bacterium—nonmotile exceptions *S. gallinarum* and *S. pullorum*, nonspore-forming and Gram-negative. There is a widespread occurrence in animals, especially in poultry and swine. Environmental sources of the organism include water, soil, insects, factory surfaces, kitchen surfaces, animal feces, raw meats, raw poultry, and raw seafoods, to name only a few.

Nature of Acute Disease

S. typhi and the paratyphoid bacteria are normally caused septicemic and produce typhoid or typhoid-like fever in humans. Other forms of salmonellosis generally produce milder symptoms.

Nature of Disease

Acute symptoms—Nausea, vomiting, abdominal cramps, minal diarrhea, fever, and headache. Chronic consequences—arthritic symptoms may follow 3-4 weeks after onset of acute symptoms.

Onset time—6-48 hours.

Foodborne Pathogenic Microorganisms and Natural Toxins Handbook, January 1992, U.S. Food & Drug Administration, Center for Food Safety & Applied Nutrition.

Infective dose—As few as 15-20 cells; depends upon age and health of host, and strain differences among the members of the genus.

Duration of symptoms—Acute symptoms may last for 1 to 2 days or may be prolonged, again depending on host factors, ingested dose, and strain characteristics.

Cause of disease—Penetration and passage of *Salmonella* organisms from gut lumen into epithelium of small intestine where inflammation occurs; there is evidence that an enterotoxin may be produced, perhaps within the enterocyte.

Diagnosis of Human Illness

Serological identification of culture isolated from stool.

Associated Foods

Raw meats, poultry, eggs, milk and dairy products, fish, shrimp, frog legs, yeast, coconut, sauces and salad dressing, cake mixes, cream-filled desserts and toppings, dried gelatin, peanut butter, cocoa, and chocolate.

Various *Salmonella* species have long been isolated from the outside of eggshells. The present situation with *S. enteritidis* is complicated by the presence of the organism inside the egg, in the yolk. This and other information strongly suggest vertical transmission, i.e., deposition of the organism in the yolk by an infected layer hen prior to shell deposition. Foods other than eggs have also caused outbreaks of *S. enteritidis* disease.

Relative Frequency of Disease

It is estimated that from 2 to 4 million cases of salmonellosis occur in the U.S. annually. The incidence of salmonellosis appears to be rising both in the U.S. and in other industrialized nations. *S. enteritidis* isolations from humans have shown a dramatic rise in the past decade, particularly in the northeast United States (6-fold or more), and the increase in human infections is spreading south and west, with sporadic outbreaks in other regions.

Complications

S. typhi and *S. paratyphi* A, B, and C produce typhoid and typhoid-like fever in humans. Various organs may be infected, leading to lesions.

The fatality rate of typhoid fever is 10% compared to less than 1% for most forms of salmonellosis. *S. dublin* has a 15% mortality rate when septicemic in the elderly, and *S. enteritidis* is demonstrating approximately a 3.6% mortality rate in hospital/nursing home outbreaks, with the elderly being particularly affected.

Salmonella septicemia has been associated with subsequent infection of virtually every organ system.

Postenteritis reactive arthritis and Reiter's syndrome have also been reported to occur generally after 3 weeks. Reactive arthritis may occur with a frequency of about 2% of culture-proven cases. Septic arthritis, subsequent or coincident with septicemia, also occurs and can be difficult to treat.

Target Populations

All age groups are susceptible, but symptoms are most severe in the elderly, infants, and the infirm. AIDS patients suffer salmonellosis frequently (estimated 20-fold more than general population) and suffer from recurrent episodes.

Foods Analysis

Methods have been developed for many foods having prior history of *Salmonella* contamination. Although conventional culture methods require 5 days for presumptive results, several rapid methods are available which require only 2 days.

Selected Outbreaks

In 1985, a salmonellosis outbreak involving 16,000 confirmed cases in 6 states was caused by low fat and whole milk from one Chicago dairy. This was the largest outbreak of foodborne salmonellosis in the U.S. FDA inspectors discovered that the pasteurization equipment had been modified to facilitate the running off of raw milk, resulting in the pasteurized milk being contaminated with raw milk under certain conditions. The dairy has subsequently disconnected the cross-linking line. Persons on antibiotic therapy were more apt to be affected in this outbreak.

In August and September, 1985, *S. enteritidis* was isolated from employees and patrons of three restaurants of a chain in Maryland. The outbreak in one restaurant had at least 71 illnesses resulting in 17 hospitalizations. Scrambled eggs from a breakfast bar were epidemiologically implicated in this outbreak and in possibly one other of the three restaurants. The plasmid profiles of isolates from patients all three restaurants matched.

The Centers for Disease Control (CDC) has recorded more than 120 outbreaks of *S. enteritidis* to date, many occurring in restaurants, and some in nursing homes, hospitals and prisons.

In 1984, 186 cases of salmonellosis (*S. enteritidis*) were reported on 29 flights to the United States on a single international airline. An estimated 2,747 passengers were affected overall. No specific food item was implicated, but food ordered from the first class menu was strongly associated with disease.

S. enteritidis outbreaks continue to occur in the U.S. The CDC estimates that 75% of those outbreaks are associated with the consumption of raw or inadequately cooked Grade A whole shell eggs. The U.S. Department of Agriculture published Regulations on February 16, 1990, in the Federal Register establishing a mandatory testing program for egg-producing breeder flocks and commercial flocks implicated in causing human illnesses. This testing should lead to a reduction in cases of gastroenteritis caused by the consumption of Grade A whole shell eggs.

Salmonellosis associated with a Thanksgiving Dinner in Nevada in 1995 is reported in *MMWR* 45(46):1996 Nov 22.

MMWR 45(34):1996 Aug 30 reports on several outbreaks of *Salmonella* enteritidis infection associated with the consumption of raw shell eggs in the United States from 1994 to 1995.

A report of an outbreak of *Salmonella* Serotype Typhimurium infection associated with the consumption of raw ground beef may be found in *MMWR* 44(49):1995 Dec 15.

MMWR 44(42):1995 Oct 27 reports on an outbreak of Salmonellosis associated with beef jerky in New Mexico in 1995.

The report on the outbreak of *Salmonella* from commercially prepared ice cream is found in *MMWR* 43(40):1994 Oct 14.

An outbreak of *S. enteritidis* in homemade ice cream is reported in *MMWR* 43(36):1994 Sep 16.

A series of *S. enteritidis* outbreaks in California are summarized in the following *MMWR* 42(41):1993 Oct 22.

For information on an outbreak of *Salmonella* Serotype Tennessee in Powdered Milk Products and Infant Formula—see *MMWR* 42(26):1993 Jul 09.

Summaries of *Salmonella* outbreaks associated with Grade A eggs are reported in *MMWR* 37(32):1988 Aug 19 and *MMWR* 39(50):1990 Dec 21.

For more information on recent outbreaks see the *Morbidity and Mortality Weekly Reports* from CDC.

Education

- The CDC provides an informational brochure on preventing *Salmonella enteritidis* infection.

- Safe Egg Handling (*FDA Consumer* Sep-Oct 1998)

Other Resources

A Loci index for genome *Salmonella enteritidis* is available from GenBank.

Chapter 13

Campylobacter

Name of the Organism

Campylobacter jejuni (formerly known as *Campylobacter fetus* subsp. jejuni). *Campylobacter jejuni* is a Gram-negative slender, curved, and motile rod. It is a microaerophilic organism, which means it has a requirement for reduced levels of oxygen. It is relatively fragile, and sensitive to environmental stresses (e.g., 21% oxygen, drying, heating, disinfectants, acidic conditions). Because of its microaerophilic characteristics the organism requires 3 to 5% oxygen and 2 to 10% carbon dioxide for optimal growth conditions. This bacterium is now recognized as an important enteric pathogen. Before 1972, when methods were developed for its isolation from feces, it was believed to be primarily an animal pathogen causing abortion and enteritis in sheep and cattle. Surveys have shown that *C. jejuni* is the leading cause of bacterial diarrheal illness in the United States. It causes more disease than *Shigella spp.* and *Salmonella spp.* combined.

Although *C. jejuni* is not carried by healthy individuals in the United States or Europe, it is often isolated from healthy cattle, chickens, birds and even flies. It is sometimes present in non-chlorinated water sources such as streams and ponds.

Because the pathogenic mechanisms of *C. jejuni* are still being studied, it is difficult to differentiate pathogenic from nonpathogenic strains. However, it appears that many of the chicken isolates are pathogens.

Foodborne Pathogenic Microorganisms and Natural Toxins Handbook, January 1992, U.S. Food & Drug Administration, Center for Food Safety & Applied Nutrition.

Name of Disease

Campylobacteriosis is the name of the illness caused by *C. jejuni*. It is also often known as campylobacter enteritis or gastroenteritis.

Major Symptoms

C. jejuni infection causes diarrhea, which may be watery or sticky and can contain blood (usually occult) and fecal leukocytes (white cells). Other symptoms often present are fever, abdominal pain, nausea, headache and muscle pain. The illness usually occurs 2-5 days after ingestion of the contaminated food or water. Illness generally lasts 7-10 days, but relapses are not uncommon (about 25% of cases). Most infections are self-limiting and are not treated with antibiotics. However, treatment with erythromycin does reduce the length of time that infected individuals shed the bacteria in their feces.

The infective dose of *C. jejuni* is considered to be small. Human feeding studies suggest that about 400-500 bacteria may cause illness in some individuals, while in others, greater numbers are required. A conducted volunteer human feeding study suggests that host susceptibility also dictates infectious dose to some degree. The pathogenic mechanisms of *C. jejuni* are still not completely understood, but it does produce a heat-labile toxin that may cause diarrhea. *C. jejuni* may also be an invasive organism.

Isolation Procedures

C. jejuni is usually present in high numbers in the diarrheal stools of individuals, but isolation requires special antibiotic-containing media and a special microaerophilic atmosphere (5% oxygen). However, most clinical laboratories are equipped to isolate *Campylobacter spp.* if requested.

Associated Foods

C. jejuni frequently contaminates raw chicken. Surveys show that 20 to 100% of retail chickens are contaminated. This is not overly surprising since many healthy chickens carry these bacteria in their intestinal tracts. Raw milk is also a source of infections. The bacteria are often carried by healthy cattle and by flies on farms. Non-chlorinated water may also be a source of infections. However, properly cooking chicken, pasteurizing milk, and chlorinating drinking water will kill the bacteria.

Frequency of the Disease

C. jejuni is the leading cause of bacterial diarrhea in the U.S. There are probably numbers of cases in excess of the estimated cases of salmonellosis (2 to 4,000,000/year).

Complications

Complications are relatively rare, but infections have been associated with reactive arthritis, hemolytic uremic syndrome, and following septicemia, infections of nearly any organ. The estimated case/fatality ratio for all *C. jejuni* infections is 0.1, meaning one death per 1,000 cases. Fatalities are rare in healthy individuals and usually occur in cancer patients or in the otherwise debilitated. Only 20 reported cases of septic abortion induced by *C. jejuni* have been recorded in the literature.

Meningitis, recurrent colitis, acute cholecystitis and Guillain-Barre syndrome are very rare complications.

Target Populations

Although anyone can have a *C. jejuni* infection, children under 5 years and young adults (15-29) are more frequently afflicted than other age groups. Reactive arthritis, a rare complication of these infections, is strongly associated with people who have the human lymphocyte antigen B27 (HLA-B27).

Recovery from Foods

Isolation of *C. jejuni* from food is difficult because the bacteria are usually present in very low numbers (unlike the case of diarrheal stools in which 10/6 bacteria/gram is not unusual). The methods require an enrichment broth containing antibiotics, special antibiotic-containing plates and a microaerophilic atmosphere generally a microaerophilic atmosphere with 5% oxygen and an elevated concentration of carbon dioxide (10%). Isolation can take several days to a week.

Selected Outbreaks

Usually outbreaks are small (less than 50 people), but in Bennington, VT a large outbreak involving about 2,000 people occurred while the town was temporarily using a non-chlorinated water source as a water supply. Several small outbreaks have been reported among children who were taken on a class trip to a dairy and given raw milk to drink. An outbreak was also associated with consumption of raw clams. However, a survey showed that about 50% of infections are associated with either eating inadequately cooked or recontaminated chicken meat or handling chickens. It is the leading bacterial cause of sporadic (non-clustered cases) diarrheal disease in the U.S.

In April, 1986, an elementary school child was cultured for bacterial pathogens (due to bloody diarrhea), and *C. jejuni* was isolated. Food consumption/gastrointestinal illness questionnaires were administered to other students and faculty at the school. In all, 32 of 172 students reported symptoms of diarrhea (100%), cramps (80%), nausea (51%), fever (29%), vomiting (26%), and bloody stools (14%). The food questionnaire clearly implicated milk as the common source, and a dose/response was evident (those drinking more milk were more likely to be ill). Investigation of the dairy supplying the milk showed that they vat pasteurized the milk at 135°F for 25 minutes rather than the required 145°F for 30 minutes. The dairy processed surplus raw milk for the school, and this milk had a high somatic cell count. Cows from the herd supplying the dairy had *C. jejuni* in their feces. This outbreak points out the variation in symptoms which may occur with campylobacteriosis and the absolute need to adhere to pasteurization time/temperature standards.

Although other *Campylobacter spp.* have been implicated in human gastroenteritis (e.g. *C. laridis*, *C. hyointestinalis*), it is believed that 99% of the cases are caused by *C. jejuni.*

For more information on recent outbreaks see the Morbidity and Mortality Weekly Reports from CDC.

Education

The Food Safety Inspection Service of the U.S. Department of Agriculture has produced a background document on Campylobacter.

Other Resources

A Loci index for genome *Campylobacter jejuni* is available from GenBank.

Chapter 14

Listeria

Name of the Organism

Listeria monocytogenes. This is a Gram-positive bacterium, motile by means of flagella. Some studies suggest that 1-10% of humans may be intestinal carriers of *L. monocytogenes*. It has been found in at least 37 mammalian species, both domestic and feral, as well as at least 17 species of birds and possibly some species of fish and shellfish. It can be isolated from soil, silage, and other environmental sources. *L. monocytogenes* is quite hardy and resists the deleterious effects of freezing, drying, and heat remarkably well for a bacterium that does not form spores. Most *L. monocytogenes* are pathogenic to some degree.

Name of Acute Disease

Listeriosis is the name of the general group of disorders caused by *L. monocytogenes*.

Nature of Disease

Listeriosis is clinically defined when the organism is isolated from blood, cerebrospinal fluid, or an otherwise normally sterile site (e.g. placenta, fetus).

Foodborne Pathogenic Microorganisms and Natural Toxins Handbook, January 1992, U.S. Food & Drug Administration, Center for Food Safety & Applied Nutrition.

The manifestations of listeriosis include septicemia, meningitis (or meningoencephalitis), encephalitis, and intrauterine or cervical infections in pregnant women, which may result in spontaneous abortion (2nd/3rd trimester) or stillbirth. The onset of the aforementioned disorders is usually preceded by influenza-like symptoms including persistent fever. It was reported that gastrointestinal symptoms such as nausea, vomiting, and diarrhea may precede more serious forms of listeriosis or may be the only symptoms expressed. Gastrointestinal symptoms were epidemiologically associated with use of antacids or cimetidine. The onset time to serious forms of listeriosis is unknown but may range from a few days to three weeks. The onset time to gastrointestinal symptoms is unknown but is probably greater than 12 hours.

The infective dose of *L. monocytogenes* is unknown but is believed to vary with the strain and susceptibility of the victim. From cases contracted through raw or supposedly pasteurized milk, it is safe to assume that in susceptible persons, fewer than 1,000 total organisms may cause disease. *L. monocytogenes* may invade the gastrointestinal epithelium. Once the bacterium enters the host's monocytes, macrophages, or polymorphonuclear leukocytes, it is bloodborne (septicemic) and can grow. Its presence intracellularly in phagocytic cells also permits access to the brain and probably transplacental migration to the fetus in pregnant women. The pathogenesis of *L. monocytogenes* centers on its ability to survive and multiply in phagocytic host cells.

Diagnosis of Human Illness

Listeriosis can only be positively diagnosed by culturing the organism from blood, cerebrospinal fluid, or stool (although the latter is difficult and of limited value).

Associated Foods

L. monocytogenes has been associated with such foods as raw milk, supposedly pasteurized fluid milk, cheeses (particularly soft-ripened varieties), ice cream, raw vegetables, fermented raw-meat sausages, raw and cooked poultry, raw meats (all types), and raw and smoked fish. Its ability to grow at temperatures as low as 30° C permits multiplication in refrigerated foods.

Frequency of the Disease

The 1987 incidence data prospectively collected by CDC suggests that there are at least 1600 cases of listeriosis with 415 deaths per year in the U.S. The vast majority of cases are sporadic, making epidemiological links to food very difficult.

Complications

Most healthy persons probably show no symptoms. The "complications" are the usual clinical expressions of the disease.

When listeric meningitis occurs, the overall mortality may be as high as 70%; from septicemia 50%, from perinatal/neonatal infections greater than 80%. In infections during pregnancy, the mother usually survives. Successful treatment with parenteral penicillin or ampicillin has been reported. Trimethoprim-sulfamethoxazole has been shown effective in patients allergic to penicillin.

Target Populations

The main target populations for listeriosis are:

- pregnant women/fetus—perinatal and neonatal infections;

- persons immunocompromised by corticosteroids, anticancer drugs,

- graft suppression therapy, AIDS;

- cancer patients—leukemic patients particularly;

- less frequently reported—diabetic, cirrhotic, asthmatic, and ulcerative colitis patients;

- the elderly;

- normal people—some reports suggest that normal, healthy people are at risk, although antacids or cimetidine may predispose. A listerosis outbreak in Switzerland involving cheese suggested that healthy uncompromised individuals could develop the disease, particularly if the foodstuff was heavily contaminated with the organism.

Food Analysis

The methods for analysis of food are complex and time consuming. The present FDA method, revised in September, 1990, requires 24 and 48 hours of enrichment, followed by a variety of other tests. Total time to identification is from 5 to 7 days, but the announcement of specific nonradiolabled DNA probes should soon allow a simpler and faster confirmation of suspect isolates.

Recombinant DNA technology may even permit 2-3 day positive analysis in the future. Currently, FDA is collaborating in adapting its methodology to quantitate very low numbers of the organisms in foods.

Selected Outbreaks

Outbreaks include the California episode in 1985, which was due to Mexican-style cheese and led to numerous stillbirths. As a result of this episode, FDA has been monitoring domestic and imported cheeses and has taken numerous actions to remove these products from the market when *L. monocytogenes* is found.

There have been other clustered cases, such as in Philadelphia, PA, in 1987. Specific food linkages were only made epidemiologically in this cluster.

CDC has established an epidemiological link between consumption of raw hot dogs or undercooked chicken and approximately 20% of the sporadic cases under prospective study.

For more information on recent outbreaks see the *Morbidity and Mortality Weekly Reports* from CDC.

Education

The FDA health alert for hispanic pregnant women concerns the risk of listeriosis from soft cheeses. The CDC provides similar information in spanish.

The Food Safety and Inspection Service of the U.S. Department of Agriculture has jointly produced with the FDA a background document on Listeria and Listeriosis. FSIS also has updated consumer information on Listeria dated February 1999.

The CDC produces an information brochure on preventing Listeriosis.

Other Resources

A Loci index for genome *Listeria monocytogenes* is available from GenBank.

Chapter 15

Bacillus

Bacillus cereus is a Gram-positive, facultatively aerobic spore-former whose cells are large rods and whose spores do not swell the sporangium. These and other characteristics, including biochemical features, are used to differentiate and confirm the presence *B. cereus*, although these characteristics are shared with *B. cereus* var. mycoides, *B. thuringiensis* and *B. anthracis*. Differentiation of these organisms depends upon determination of motility (most *B. cereus* are motile), presence of toxin crystals (*B. thuringiensis*), hemolytic activity (*B. cereus* and others are beta hemolytic whereas *B. anthracis* is usually nonhemolytic), and rhizoid growth which is characteristic of *B. cereus* var. mycoides.

Name of Illness

B. cercus food poisoning is the general description, although two recognized types of illness are caused by two distinct metabolites. The diarrheal type of illness is caused by a large molecular weight protein, while the vomiting (emetic) type of illness is believed to be caused by a low molecular weight, heat-stable peptide.

Foodborne Pathogenic Microorganisms and Natural Toxins Handbook, January 1992, U.S. Food & Drug Administration, Center for Food Safety & Applied Nutrition.

Nature of Illness

The symptoms of *B. cereus* diarrheal type food poisoning mimic those of *Clostridium perfringens* food poisoning. The onset of watery diarrhea, abdominal cramps, and pain occurs 6-15 hours after consumption of contaminated food. Nausea may accompany diarrhea, but vomiting (emesis) rarely occurs. Symptoms persist for 24 hours in most instances.

The emetic type of food poisoning is characterized by nausea and vomiting within 0.5 to 6 h after consumption of contaminated foods. Occasionally, abdominal cramps and/or diarrhea may also occur. Duration of symptoms is generally less than 24 h. The symptoms of this type of food poisoning parallel those caused by *Staphylococcus aureus* foodborne intoxication. Some strains of *B. subtilis* and *B. licheniformis* have been isolated from lamb and chicken incriminated in food poisoning episodes. These organisms demonstrate the production of a highly heat-stable toxin which may be similar to the vomiting type toxin produced by *B. cereus*.

The presence of large numbers of *B. cereus* (greater than 10^6 organisms/g) in a food is indicative of active growth and proliferation of the organism and is consistent with a potential hazard to health.

Diagnosis of Human Illness

Confirmation of *B. cereus* as the etiologic agent in a foodborne outbreak requires either (1) isolation of strains of the same serotype from the suspect food and feces or vomitus of the patient, (2) isolation of large numbers of a *B. cereus* serotype known to cause foodborne illness from the suspect food or from the feces or vomitus of the patient, or (3) isolation of *B. cereus* from suspect foods and determining their enterotoxigenicity by serological (diarrheal toxin) or biological (diarrheal and emetic) tests. The rapid onset time to symptoms in the emetic form of disease, coupled with some food evidence, is often sufficient to diagnose this type of food poisoning.

Foods Incriminated

A wide variety of foods including meats, milk, vegetables, and fish have been associated with the diarrheal type food poisoning. The vomiting-type outbreaks have generally been associated with rice products; however, other starchy foods such as potato, pasta and cheese products have also been implicated. Food mixtures such as sauces, puddings, soups, casseroles, pastries, and salads have frequently been incriminated in food poisoning outbreaks.

Relative Frequency of Illness

In 1980, 9 outbreaks were reported to the Centers for Disease Control and included such foods as beef, turkey, and Mexican foods. In 1981, 8 outbreaks were reported which primarily involved rice and shellfish. Other outbreaks go unreported or are misdiagnosed because of symptomatic similarities to *Staphylococcus aureus* intoxication *(B. cereus* vomiting-type) or *C. perfringens* food poisoning (*B. cereus* diarrheal type).

Complications

Although no specific complications have been associated with the diarrheal and vomiting toxins produced by *B. cereus*, other clinical manifestations of *B. cereus* invasion or contamination have been observed. They include bovine mastitis, severe systemic and pyogenic infections, gangrene, septic meningitis, cellulitis, panophthalmitis, lung abscesses, infant death, and endocarditis.

Target Populations

All people are believed to be susceptible to *B. cereus* food poisoning.

Food Analysis

A variety of methods have been recommended for the recovery, enumeration and confirmation of B. cereus in foods. More recently, a serological method has been developed for detecting the putative enterotoxin of *B. cereus* (diarrheal type) isolates from suspect foods. Recent investigations suggest that the vomiting type toxin can be detected by animal models (cats, monkeys) or possibly by cell culture.

Selected Outbreaks

On September 22, 1985, the Maine Bureau of Health was notified of gastrointestinal illness among patrons of a Japanese restaurant. Because the customers were exhibiting symptoms of illness while still on the restaurant premises, and because uncertainty existed as to the etiology of the problem, the local health department, in concurrence with the restaurant owner, closed the restaurant at 7:30 p.m. that same day.

Eleven (31%) of the approximately 36 patrons reportedly served on the evening of September 22, were contacted in an effort to determine the etiology of the outbreak. Those 11 comprised the last three dining parties served on September 22. Despite extensive publicity, no additional cases were reported.

A case was defined as anyone who demonstrated vomiting or diarrhea within 6 hours of dining at the restaurant. All 11 individuals were interviewed for symptoms, time of onset of illness, illness duration, and foods ingested. All 11 reported nausea and vomiting; nine reported diarrhea; one reported headache; and one reported abdominal cramps. Onset of illness ranged from 30 minutes to 5 hours (mean 1 hour, 23 minutes) after eating at the restaurant. Duration of illness ranged from 5 hours to several days, except for two individuals still symptomatic with diarrhea 2 weeks after dining at the restaurant. Ten persons sought medical treatment at local emergency rooms on September 22; two ultimately required hospitalization for rehydration.

Analysis of the association of specific foods with illness was not instructive, since all persons consumed the same food items; chicken soup, fried shrimp, stir-fried rice, fried zucchini, onions, bean sprouts, cucumber, cabbage, and lettuce salad, ginger salad dressing, hibachi chicken and steak, and tea. Five persons ordered hibachi scallops, and one person ordered hibachi swordfish. However, most individuals sampled each other's entrees. One vomitus specimen and two stool specimens from the three separate individuals yielded an overgrowth of *B. cereus*, although an accurate bacterial count could not be made because an inadequate amount of the steak remained for laboratory analysis. No growth of *B. cereus* was reported from the fried rice, mixed fried vegetables, or hibachi chicken.

According to the owner, all meat was delivered 2-3 times a week from a local meat supplier and refrigerated until ordered by restaurant patrons. Appropriate-sized portions for a dining group were taken from the kitchen to the dining area and diced or sliced, then sauteed at the table directly in front of restaurant patrons. The meat was seasoned with soy sauce salt and white pepper, open containers of which had been used for at least 2 months by the restaurant. The hibachi steak was served immediately after cooking.

The fried rice served with the meal was customarily made from leftover boiled rice. It could not be established whether the boiled rice had been stored refrigerated or at room temperature.

Fresh, rapidly cooked meat, eaten immediately, seems an unlikely vehicle of *B. cereus* food poisoning. The laboratory finding of *B. cereus* in a foodstuff without quantitative cultures and without accompanying epidemiologic data is insufficient to establish its role in the outbreak. Although no viable *B. cereus* organisms were isolated from the fried rice eaten with the meal, it does not exclude this food as the common vehicle. Reheating during preparation may have eliminated the bacteria in the food without decreasing the activity of the heat-stable toxin. While the question of the specific vehicle remains incompletely resolved, the clinical and laboratory findings substantially support *B. cereus* as the cause of the outbreak.

Most episodes of food poisoning undoubtedly go unreported, and in most of those reported, the specific pathogens are never identified. Alert recognition of the clinical syndrome and appropriate laboratory work permitted identification of the role of *B. cereus* in this outbreak.

Updates

For a report on a *B. cereus* outbreak in northern Virginia see *MMWR* 43(10):1994 Mar 18.

For more information on recent outbreaks see the *Morbidity and Mortality Weekly Reports* from CDC.

Chapter 16

Plesiomonas Shigelloides

Name of the Organism

Plesiomonas shigelloides is a Gram-negative, rod-shaped bacterium which has been isolated from freshwater, freshwater fish, and shellfish and from many types of animals including cattle, goats, swine, cats, dogs, monkeys, vultures, snakes, and toads.

Most human *P. shigelloides* infections are suspected to be waterborne. The organism may be present in unsanitary water which has been used as drinking water, recreational water, or water used to rinse foods that are consumed without cooking or heating. The ingested *P. shigelloides* organism does not always cause illness in the host animal but may reside temporarily as a transient, noninfectious member of the intestinal flora. It has been isolated from the stools of patients with diarrhea, but is also sometimes isolated from healthy individuals (0.2-3.2% of population).

It cannot yet be considered a definite cause of human disease, although its association with human diarrhea and the virulence factors it demonstrates make it a prime candidate.

Name of Acute Disease

Gastroenteritis is the disease with which *P. shigelloides* has been implicated.

Foodborne Pathogenic Microorganisms and Natural Toxins Handbook, January 1992, U.S. Food & Drug Administration, Center for Food Safety & Applied Nutrition.

Nature of Disease

P. shigelloides gastroenteritis is usually a mild self-limiting disease with fever, chills, abdominal pain, nausea, diarrhea, or vomiting; symptoms may begin 20-24 hours after consumption of contaminated food or water; diarrhea is watery, non-mucoid, and non-bloody; in severe cases, diarrhea may be greenish-yellow, foamy, and blood tinged; duration of illness in healthy people may be 1-7 days.

The infectious dose is presumed to be quite high, at least greater than one million organisms.

Diagnosis of Human Illness

The pathogenesis of *P. shigelloides* infection is not known. The organism is suspected of being toxigenic and invasive. Its significance as an enteric (intestinal) pathogen is presumed because of its predominant isolation from stools of patients with diarrhea. It is identified by common bacteriological analysis, serotyping, and antibiotic sensitivity testing.

Associated Foods

Most *P. shigelloides* infections occur in the summer months and correlate with environmental contamination of freshwater (rivers, streams, ponds, etc.). The usual route of transmission of the organism in sporadic or epidemic cases is by ingestion of contaminated water or raw shellfish.

Frequency of Disease

Most *P. shigelloides* strains associated with human gastrointestinal disease have been from stools of diarrheic patients living in tropical and subtropical areas. Such infections are rarely reported in the U.S. or Europe because of the self-limiting nature of the disease.

Usual Course of Disease and Some Complications

P. shigelloides infection may cause diarrhea of 1-2 days duration in healthy adults. However, there may be high fever and chills and protracted dysenteric symptoms in infants and children under 15 years of age. Extra-intestinal complications (septicemia and death) may occur in people who are immunocompromised or seriously ill with cancer, blood disorders, or hepatobiliary disease.

Target Populations

All people may be susceptible to infection. Infants, children and chronically ill people are more likely to experience protracted illness and complications.

Food Analysis

P. shigelloides may be recovered from food and water by methods similar to those used for stool analysis. The keys to recovery in all cases are selective agars which enhance the survival and growth of these bacteria over the growth of the background microflora. Identification following recovery may be completed in 12-24 hours.

Selected Outbreaks

Gastrointestinal illness in healthy people caused by *P. shigelloides* infection may be so mild that they do not seek medical treatment. Its rate of occurrence in the U.S. is unknown. It may be included in the group of diarrheal diseases "of unknown etiology" which are treated with and respond to broad spectrum antibiotics.

Most cases reported in the United States involve individuals with preexisting health problems such as cancer, sickle cell anemia, immunoincompetence, the aged, and the very young, who develop complications.

A case cluster occurred in North Carolina in November, 1980, following an oyster roast. Thirty-six out of 150 people who had eaten roasted oysters experienced nausea, chills, fever, vomiting, diarrhea, and abdominal pain beginning 2 days after the roast. The average duration of these symptoms was 2 days. *P. shigelloides* was recovered from oyster samples and patient stools.

A non-food related outbreak of *P. shigelloides* is reported in *MMWR* 38(36):1989 Sep 15.

For more information on recent outbreaks see the *Morbidity and Mortality Weekly Reports* from CDC.

Chapter 17

Shigella

Name of the Organism

Shigella spp. (*Shigella sonnei, S. boydii, S. flexneri,* and *S. dysenteriae*). *Shigella* are Gram-negative, nonmotile, nonsporeforming rod-shaped bacteria. The illness caused by *Shigella* (shigellosis) accounts for less than 10% of the reported outbreaks of foodborne illness in this country. *Shigella* rarely occurs in animals; principally a disease of humans except other primates such as monkeys and chimpanzees. The organism is frequently found in water polluted with human feces.

Name of Disease

Shigellosis (bacillary dysentery).

Nature of Disease

Symptoms—Abdominal pain; cramps; diarrhea; fever; vomiting; blood, pus, or mucus in stools; tenesmus.

Onset time—12 to 50 hours.

Infective dose—As few as 10 cells depending on age and condition of host. The *Shigella* spp. are highly infectious agents that are transmitted by the fecal-oral route.

Foodborne Pathogenic Microorganisms and Natural Toxins Handbook, January 1992, U.S. Food & Drug Administration, Center for Food Safety & Applied Nutrition.

The disease is caused when virulent *Shigella* organisms attach to, and penetrate, epithelial cells of the intestinal mucosa. After invasion, they multiply intracellularly, and spread to contiguous epitheleal cells resulting in tissue destruction. Some strains produce enterotoxin and Shiga toxin (very much like the verotoxin of *E. coli* O157:H7).

Diagnosis of Human Illness

Serological identification of culture isolated from stool.

Associated Foods

Salads (potato, tuna, shrimp, macaroni, and chicken), raw vegetables, milk and dairy products, and poultry. Contamination of these foods is usually through the fecal-oral route. Fecally contaminated water and unsanitary handling by food handlers are the most common causes of contamination.

Relative Frequency of Disease

An estimated 300,000 cases of shigellosis occur annually in the U.S. The number attributable to food is unknown, but given the low infectious dose, it is probably substantial.

Complications

Infections are associated with mucosal ulceration, rectal bleeding, drastic dehydration; fatality may be as high as 10-15% with some strains. Reiter's disease, reactive arthritis, and hemolytic uremic syndrome are possible sequelae that have been reported in the aftermath of shigellosis.

Target Populations

Infants, the elderly, and the infirm are susceptible to the severest symptoms of disease, but all humans are susceptible to some degree. Shigellosis is a very common malady suffered by individuals with acquired immune deficiency syndrome (AIDS) and AIDS-related complex, as well as non-AIDS homosexual men.

Food Analysis

Organisms are difficult to demonstrate in foods because methods are not developed or are insensitive. A genetic probe to the virulence plasmid has been developed by FDA and is currently under field test. However, the isolation procedures are still poor.

Selected Outbreaks

In 1985, a huge outbreak of foodborne shigellosis occurred in Midland-Odessa, Texas, involving perhaps as many as 5,000 persons. The implicated food was chopped, bagged lettuce, prepared in a central location for a Mexican restaurant chain. FDA research subsequently showed that *S. sonnei*, the isolate from the lettuce, could survive in chopped lettuce under refrigeration, and the lettuce remained fresh and appeared to be quite edible.

In 1985-1986, several outbreaks of shigellosis occurred on college campuses, usually associated with fresh vegetables from the salad bar. Usually an ill food service worker was shown to be the cause. In 1987, several very large outbreaks of shigellosis (*S. sonnei*) occurred involving thousands of persons, but no specific food vector could be proven.

In 1988, numerous individuals contracted shigellosis from food consumed aboard Northwest Airlines flights; food on these flights had been prepared in one central commissary. No specific food item was implicated, but various sandwiches were suspected.

Although all *Shigella* spp. have been implicated in foodborne outbreaks at some time, *S. sonnei* is clearly the leading cause of shigellosis from food. The other species are more closely associated with contaminated water. One in particular, *S. flexneri*, is now thought to be in large part sexually transmitted.

For information on the outbreak of *Shigella* on a cruise ship, see *MMWR* 43(35):1994 Sep 09

MMWR 40(25):1991 Jun 28 reports on a *Shigella dysenteriae* Type 1 outbreak in Guatemala, 1991.

For more information on recent outbreaks see the *Morbidity and Mortality Weekly Reports* from CDC.

Chapter 18

Streptococcus

Name of the Organism

The genus *Streptococcus* is comprised of Gram-positive, microaerophilic cocci (round), which are not motile and occur in chains or pairs. The genus is defined by a combination of antigenic, hemolytic, and physiological characteristics into Groups A, B, C, D, F, and G. Groups A and D can be transmitted to humans via food.

Group A: one species with 40 antigenic types (S. *pyogenes*).

Group D: five species (*S. faecalis*, *S. faecium*, *S. durans*, *S. avium*, and *S. bovis*).

Name of Acute Disease

Group A: Cause septic sore throat and scarlet fever as well as other pyogenic and septicemic infections.

Group D: May produce a clinical syndrome similar to staphylococcal intoxication.

Nature of Illness/Disease

Group A: Sore and red throat, pain on swallowing, tonsilitis, high fever, headache, nausea, vomiting, malaise, rhinorrhea; occasionally

Foodborne Pathogenic Microorganisms and Natural Toxins Handbook, January 1992, U.S. Food & Drug Administration, Center for Food Safety & Applied Nutrition.

a rash occurs, onset 1-3 days; the infectious dose is probably quite low (less than 1,000 organisms).

Group D: Diarrhea, abdominal cramps, nausea, vomiting, fever, chills, dizziness in 2-36 hours. Following ingestion of suspect food, the infectious dose is probably high (greater than 107 organisms).

Diagnosis of Human Disease

Group A: Culturing of nasal and throat swabs, pus, sputum, blood, suspect food, environmental samples.

Group D: Culturing of stool samples, blood, and suspect food.

Associated Foods

Group A: Food sources include milk, ice cream, eggs, steamed lobster, ground ham, potato salad, egg salad, custard, rice pudding, and shrimp salad. In almost all cases, the foodstuffs were allowed to stand at room temperature for several hours between preparation and consumption. Entrance into the food is the result of poor hygiene, ill food handlers, or the use of unpasteurized milk.

Group D: Food sources include sausage, evaporated milk, cheese, meat croquettes, meat pie, pudding, raw milk, and pasteurized milk. Entrance into the food chain is due to underprocessing and/or poor and unsanitary food preparation.

Relative Frequency of Infection

Group A infections are low and may occur in any season, whereas Group D infections are variable.

Usual Course of Disease and Complications

Group A: Streptococcal sore throat is very common, especially in children. Usually it is successfully treated with antibiotics. Complications are rare and the fatality rate is low.

Group D: Diarrheal illness is poorly characterized, but is acute and self-limiting.

Target Population

All individuals are susceptible. No age or race susceptibilities have been found.

Analysis of Foods

Suspect food is examined microbiologically by selective enumeration techniques which can take up to 7 days. Group specificities are determined by Lancefield group-specific antisera.

Selected Outbreaks

Group A: Outbreaks of septic sore throat and scarlet fever were numerous before the advent of milk pasteurization. Salad bars have been suggested as possible sources of infection. Most current outbreaks have involved complex foods (i.e., salads) which were infected by a food handler with septic sore throat. One ill food handler may subsequently infect hundreds of individuals.

Group D: Outbreaks are not common and are usually the result of preparing, storing, or handling food in an unsanitary manner.

For more information on recent outbreaks see the *Morbidity and Mortality Weekly Reports* from CDC.

Chapter 19

Enterotoxigenic Escherichia Coli

Name of the Organism

Enterotoxigenic *Escherichia coli* (ETEC). Currently, there are four recognized classes of enterovirulent *E. coli* (collectively referred to as the EEC group) that cause gastroenteritis in humans. Among these are the enterotoxigenic (ETEC) strains. They comprise a relatively small proportion of the species and have been etiologically associated with diarrheal illness of all age groups from diverse global locations. The organism frequently causes diarrhea in infants in less developed countries and in visitors there from industrialized countries. The etiology of this cholera-like illness has been recognized for about 20 years.

Name of Acute Disease

Gastroenteritis is the common name of the illness caused by ETEC, although travelers' diarrhea is a frequent sobriquet.

Nature of Disease

The most frequent clinical syndrome of infection includes watery diarrhea, abdominal cramps, low-grade fever, nausea and malaise.

Foodborne Pathogenic Microorganisms and Natural Toxins Handbook, January 1992, U.S. Food & Drug Administration, Center for Food Safety & Applied Nutrition.

Infective dose—Volunteer feeding studies indicate that a relatively large dose (100 million to 10 billion bacteria) of enterotoxigenic *E. coli* is probably necessary to establish colonization of the small intestine, where these organisms proliferate and produce toxins which induce fluid secretion. With high infective dose, diarrhea can be induced within 24 hours. Infants may require fewer organisms for infection to be established.

Diagnosis of Human Illness

During the acute phase of infection, large numbers of enterotoxigenic cells are excreted in feces. These strains are differentiated from nontoxigenic *E. coli* present in the bowel by a variety of in vitro immunochemical, tissue culture, or gene probe tests designed to detect either the toxins or genes that encode for these toxins. The diagnosis can be completed in about 3 days.

Associated Foods

ETEC is not considered a serious foodborne disease hazard in countries having high sanitary standards and practices. Contamination of water with human sewage may lead to contamination of foods. Infected food handlers may also contaminate foods. These organisms are infrequently isolated from dairy products such as semi-soft cheeses.

Relative Frequency of Disease

Only four outbreaks in the U.S. have been documented, one resulting from consumption of water contaminated with human sewage, another from consumption of Mexican food prepared by an infected food handler. In two others, one in a hospital cafeteria and one aboard a cruise ship, food was the probable cause. The disease among travelers to foreign countries, however, is common.

Complications

The disease is usually self-limiting. In infants or debilitated elderly persons, appropriate electrolyte replacement therapy may be necessary.

Target Populations

Infants and travelers to underdeveloped countries are most at-risk of infection.

Analysis of Food

With the availability of a gene probe method, foods can be analyzed directly for the presence of enterotoxigenic *E. coli*, and the analysis can be completed in about 3 days. Alternative methods which involve enrichment and plating of samples for isolation of *E. coli* and their subsequent confirmation as toxigenic strains by conventional toxin assays may take at least 7 days.

Selected Outbreaks

In the last decade, four major common-source outbreaks of ETEC gastroenteritis occurred in the U.S. In late 1975 one-third of the passengers on two successive cruises of a Miami-based ship experienced diarrheal illness. A CDC investigation found ETEC to be the cause, presumably linked to consumption of crabmeat cocktail. In early 1980, 415 persons eating at a Mexican restaurant experienced diarrhea. The source of the causative organism was an ill food handler. In 1981, 282 of 3,000 personnel at a Texas hospital acquired ETEC gastroenteritis after eating in the hospital cafeteria. No single food was identified by CDC.

Outbreaks of ETEC in Rhode Island and New Hampshire are reported in this MMWR 43(5):1994 Feb 11.

Chapter 20

Enteropathogenic Escherichia Coli

Name of the Organism

Enteropathogenic *Escherichia coli* (EPEC). Currently, there are four recognized classes of enterovirulent *E. coli* (collectively referred to as the EEC group) that cause gastroenteritis in humans. Among these are the enteropathogenic (EPEC) strains. EPEC are defined as *E. coli* belonging to serogroups epidemiologically implicated as pathogens but whose virulence mechanism is unrelated to the excretion of typical *E. coli* enterotoxins. *E. coli* are Gram-negative, rod-shaped bacteria belonging the family Enterobacteriaceae. Source(s) and prevalence of EPEC are controversial because foodborne outbreaks are sporadic. Humans, bovines, and swine can be infected, and the latter often serve as common experimental animal models. *E. coli* are present in the normal gut flora of these mammals. The proportion of pathogenic to nonpathogenic strains, although the subject of intense research, is unknown.

Name of Acute Disease

Infantile diarrhea is the name of the disease usually associated with EPEC.

Foodborne Pathogenic Microorganisms and Natural Toxins Handbook, January 1992, U.S. Food & Drug Administration, Center for Food Safety & Applied Nutrition.

Nature of Disease

EPEC cause either a watery or bloody diarrhea, the former associated with the attachment to, and physical alteration of, the integrity of the intestine. Bloody diarrhea is associated with attachment and an acute tissue-destructive process, perhaps caused by a toxin similar to that of *Shigella dysenteriae*, also called verotoxin. In most of these strains the shiga-like toxin is cell-associated rather than excreted.

Infective dose—EPEC are highly infectious for infants and the dose is presumably very low. In the few documented cases of adult diseases, the dose is presumably similar to other colonizers (greater than 10^6 total dose).

Diagnosis of Human Illness

The distinction of EPEC from other groups of pathogenic *E. coli* isolated from patients' stools involves serological and cell culture assays. Serotyping, although useful, is not strict for EPEC.

Associated Foods

Common foods implicated in EPEC outbreaks are raw beef and chicken, although any food exposed to fecal contamination is strongly suspect.

Relative Frequency of Disease

Outbreaks of EPEC are sporadic. Incidence varies on a worldwide basis; countries with poor sanitation practices have the most frequent outbreaks.

Usual Course of Disease and Some Complications

Occasionally, diarrhea in infants is prolonged, leading to dehydration, electrolyte imbalance and death (50% mortality rates have been reported in third world countries).

Target Populations

EPEC outbreaks most often affect infants, especially those that are bottle fed, suggesting that contaminated water is often used to rehydrate infant formulae in underdeveloped countries.

Analysis of Foods

The isolation and identification of *E. coli* in foods follows standard enrichment and biochemical procedures. Serotyping of isolates to distinguish EPEC is laborious and requires high quality, specific antisera, and technical expertise. The total analysis may require from 7 to 14 days.

Selected Outbreaks

Sporadic outbreaks of EPEC diarrhea have occurred for half a century in infant nurseries, presumably derived from the hospital environment or contaminated infant formula. Common-source outbreaks of EPEC diarrhea involving healthy young adults were reported in the late 1960s. Presumably a large inoculum was ingested.

Chapter 21

Escherichia Coli *O157:H7*

Name of the Organism

Escherichia coli O157:H7 (enterohemorrhagic *E. coli* or EHEC). Currently, there are four recognized classes of enterovirulent *E. coli* (collectively referred to as the EEC group) that cause gastroenteritis in humans. Among these is the enterohemorrhagic (EHEC) strain designated *E. coli* O157:H7. *E. coli* is a normal inhabitant of the intestines of all animals, including humans. When aerobic culture methods are used, *E. coli* is the dominant species found in feces. Normally *E. coli* serves a useful function in the body by suppressing the growth of harmful bacterial species and by synthesizing appreciable amounts of vitamins. A minority of *E. coli* strains are capable of causing human illness by several different mechanisms. *E. coli* serotype O157:H7 is a rare variety of *E. coli* that produces large quantities of one or more related, potent toxins that cause severe damage to the lining of the intestine. These toxins [verotoxin (VT), shiga-like toxin] are closely related or identical to the toxin produced by *Shigella* dysenteriae.

Name of Acute Disease

Hemorrhagic colitis is the name of the acute disease caused by *E. coli* O157:H7.

Foodborne Pathogenic Microorganisms and Natural Toxins Handbook, January 1992, U.S. Food & Drug Administration, Center for Food Safety & Applied Nutrition.

Nature of Disease

The illness is characterized by severe cramping (abdominal pain) and diarrhea which is initially watery but becomes grossly bloody. Occasionally vomiting occurs. Fever is either low-grade or absent. The illness is usually self-limited and lasts for an average of 8 days. Some individuals exhibit watery diarrhea only.

Infective dose—Unknown, but from a compilation of outbreak data, including the organism's ability to be passed person-to-person in the day-care setting and nursing homes, the dose may be similar to that of *Shigella* spp. (10 organisms).

Diagnosis of Human Illness

Hemorrhagic colitis is diagnosed by isolation of *E. coli* of serotype O157:H7 or other verotoxin-producing *E. coli* from diarrheal stools. Alternatively, the stools can be tested directly for the presence of verotoxin. Confirmation can be obtained by isolation of *E. coli* of the same serotype from the incriminated food.

Associated Foods

Undercooked or raw hamburger (ground beef) has been implicated in nearly all documented outbreaks and in other sporadic cases. Raw milk was the vehicle in a school outbreak in Canada. These are the only two demonstrated food causes of disease, but other meats may contain *E. coli* O157:H7.

Relative Frequency of Disease

Hemorrhagic colitis infections are not too common, but this is probably not reflective of the true frequency. In the Pacific Northwest, *E. coli* O157:H7 is thought to be second only to Salmonella as a cause of bacterial diarrhea. Because of the unmistakable symptoms of profuse, visible blood in severe cases, those victims probably seek medical attention, but less severe cases are probably more numerous.

Usual Course of Disease and Some Complications

Some victims, particularly the very young, have developed the hemolytic uremic syndrome (HUS), characterized by renal failure and hemolytic anemia. From 0 to 15% of hemorrhagic colitis victims may develop HUS. The disease can lead to permanent loss of kidney function. In the elderly, HUS, plus two other symptoms, fever and neurologic symptoms, constitutes thrombotic thrombocytopenic purpura (TTP). This illness can have a mortality rate in the elderly as high as 50%.

Target Populations

All people are believed to be susceptible to hemorrhagic colitis, but larger outbreaks have occurred in institutional settings.

Analysis of Foods

E. coli 0157:H7 will form colonies on agar media that are selective for *E. coli*. However, the high temperature growth procedure normally performed to eliminate background organisms before plating cannot be used because of the inability of these organisms to grow at temperatures of 44.0 - 45.5°C that support the growth of most *E. coli*. The use of DNA probes to detect genes encoding for the production of verotoxins (VT1 and VT2) is the most sensitive method devised.

Selected Outbreaks

Three outbreaks occurred in 1982. Two of them, one in Michigan and one in Oregon, involved hamburgers from a national fast-food chain. The third occurred in a home for the aged in Ottawa, Ontario; club sandwiches were implicated, and 19 people died. More recently, several outbreaks in nursing homes and a day-care center have been investigated. Two large outbreaks occurred in 1984, one in 1985, three in 1986. Larger outbreaks have occurred in the Northwest U.S. and Canada.

In October-November, 1986, an outbreak of hemorrhagic colitis caused by *E. coli* 0157:H7 occurred in Walla Walla, WA. Thirty-seven people, aged 11 months to 78 years developed diarrhea caused by the organism. All isolates from patients (14) had a unique plasmid profile and produced Shiga-like toxin II. In addition to diarrhea, 36 persons reported grossly bloody stools and 36 of the 37 reported abdominal cramps. Seventeen patients were hospitalized. One patient developed HUS (4 years old) and three developed TTP (70, 78, and 78 years old). Two patients with TTP died. Ground beef was the implicated food vehicle.

An excellent summary of nine *E. coli* 0157:H7 outbreaks appeared in the Annals of Internal Medicine, 1 November, 1988, pp.

705-712. There was a recall of frozen hamburger underway (12 Aug 1997). For more information, see the USDA announcement and follow-up announcement (15 Aug 1997) on the U.S. Department of Agriculture web site concerning the recall of Hudson frozen ground beef.

The Centers for Disease Control and Prevention have reported on the above outbreak in preliminary (*MMWR* 45(44):975, 1996 November 8) and in updated (*MMWR* 46(1):4-8, 1997 January 10) form.

The FDA has issued on 31 October 1996 a press release concerning an outbreak of *E. coli* O157:H7 associated with Odwalla brand apple juice products.

A non-food related outbreak of *E. coli* O157:H7 is reported in *MMWR* 45(21):1996 May 31. While, the source of the outbreak is thought to be waterborne, the article is linked to this chapter to provide updated reference information on enterohemorrhagic *E. coli*. *MMWR* 45(12):1996 Mar 29 reports on an outbreak of O157:H7 that occured in Georgia and Tennessee in June of 1995.

A community outbreak of hemolytic uremic syndrome attributable to *Escherichia coli* O111:NM in southern Australia in 1995 is reported in *MMWR* 44(29):1995 Jul 28.

A report on enhanced detection of sporadic *E. coli* O157:H7 infections in New Jersey and on an *E. coli* O157:H7 outbreak at a summer camp are in *MMWR* 44(22): 1995 Jun 9.

An outbreak of *E. coli* O157:H7 in Washington and California associated with dry-cured salami is reported in *MMWR* 44(9):1995 Mar 10.

Information concerning an outbreak that occured because of home-cooked hamburger can be found in this *MMWR* 43(12):1994 Apr 01. *MMWR* 43(10):1994 Mar 18 reports on laboratory screening for *E. coli* O157 in Connecticut.

The outbreak of EHEC in the western states of the US is reported in preliminary form in this *MMWR* 42(4):1993 Feb 5, and in updated form in this *MMWR* 42(14):1993 Apr 16.

An outbreak of *E. coli* O157 in 1990 in North Dakota is reported in the *MMWR* 40(16):1991 Apr 26.

The Centers for Disease Control and Prevention has reissued the 5 November 1982 *MMWR* report that was the first to describe the diarrheal illness of *E. coli* O157:H7. This reissue is a part of the commemoration of CDC's 50th anniversary.

For more information on recent outbreaks see the *Morbidity and Mortality Weekly Reports* from CDC.

Education

USDA Urges Consumers To Use Food Thermometer When Cooking Ground Beef Patties (Aug 11 1998).

The CDC has an information brochure on preventing *Escherichia coli* O157:H7 infections.

Other Resources

Dr. Feng of FDA/CFSAN has written a monograph on *E. coli* O157:H7 which appeared in the CDC journal Emerging Infectious Diseases Vol. 1 No. 2, April-June 1995.

Chapter 22

Enteroinvasive Escherichia Coli

Name of the Organism

Enteroinvasive *Escherichia coli* or (EIEC). Currently, there are four recognized classes of enterovirulent *E. coli* (collectively referred to as the EEC group) that cause gastroenteritis in humans. *E. coli* is part of the normal intestinal flora of humans and other primates. A minority of *E. coli* strains are capable of causing human illness by several different mechanisms. Among these are the enteroinvasive (EIEC) strains. It is unknown what foods may harbor these pathogenic enteroinvasive (EIEC) strains responsible for a form of bacillary dysentery.

Name of Disease

Enteroinvasive *E. coli* (EIEC) may produce an illness known as bacillary dysentery. The EIEC strains responsible for this syndrome are closely related to *Shigella* spp.

Nature of the Disease

Following the ingestion of EIEC, the organisms invade the epithelial cells of the intestine, resulting in a mild form of dysentery, often

Foodborne Pathogenic Microorganisms and Natural Toxins Handbook, January 1992, U.S. Food & Drug Administration, Center for Food Safety & Applied Nutrition.

mistaken for dysentery caused by *Shigella* species. The illness is characterized by the appearance of blood and mucus in the stools of infected individuals.

Infective dose—The infectious dose of EIEC is thought to be as few as 10 organisms (same as *Shigella*).

Diagnosis of Human Illness

The culturing of the organism from the stools of infected individuals and the demonstration of invasiveness of isolates in tissue culture or in a suitable animal model is necessary to diagnose dysentery caused by this organism.

More recently, genetic probes for the invasiveness genes of both EIEC and *Shigella* spp. have been developed.

Associated Foods

It is currently unknown what foods may harbor EIEC, but any food contaminated with human feces from an ill individual, either directly or via contaminated water, could cause disease in others. Outbreaks have been associated with hamburger meat and unpasteurized milk.

Relative Frequency of Disease

One major foodborne outbreak attributed to enteroinvasive *E. coli* in the U.S. occurred in 1973. It was due to the consumption of imported cheese from France. The disease caused by EIEC is uncommon, but it may be confused with shigellosis and its prevalence may be underestimated.

The Usual Course of Disease and Some Complications

Dysentery caused by EIEC usually occurs within 12 to 72 hours following the ingestion of contaminated food. The illness is characterized by abdominal cramps, diarrhea, vomiting, fever, chills, and a generalized malaise. Dysentery caused by this organism is generally self-limiting with no known complications. A common sequelus associated with infection, especially in pediatric cases, is hemolytic uremic syndrome (HUS).

Target Populations

All people are subject to infection by this organism.

Analysis of Foods

Foods are examined as are stool cultures. Detection of this organism in foods is extremely difficult because undetectable levels may cause illness. It is estimated that the ingestion of as few as 10 organisms may result in dysentery.

Selected Outbreaks

Several outbreaks in the U.S. have been attributed to this organism. One outbreak occurred in 1973 and was due to the consumption of imported cheese. More recently, a cruise ship outbreak was attributed to potato salad, and an outbreak occurred in a home for the mentally retarded where subsequent person-to-person transmission occurred.

Chapter 23

Giardia Lamblia

Name of the Organism

Giardia lamblia (intestinalis) is a single celled animal, i.e., a protozoa, that moves with the aid of five flagella. In Europe, it is sometimes referred to as Lamblia intestinalis.

Disease Name

Giardiasis is the most frequent cause of non-bacterial diarrhea in North America.

Nature of the Disease

Organisms that appear identical to those that cause human illness have been isolated from domestic animals (dogs and cats) and wild animals (beavers and bears). A related but morphologically distinct organism infects rodents, although rodents may be infected with human isolates in the laboratory. Human giardiasis may involve diarrhea within 1 week of ingestion of the cyst, which is the environmental survival form and infective stage of the organism. Normally illness lasts for 1 to 2 weeks, but there are cases of chronic infections lasting months to years. Chronic cases, both those with defined immune

Foodborne Pathogenic Microorganisms and Natural Toxins Handbook, January 1992, U.S. Food & Drug Administration, Center for Food Safety & Applied Nutrition.

deficiencies and those without, are difficult to treat. The disease mechanism is unknown, with some investigators reporting that the organism produces a toxin while others are unable to confirm its existence. The organism has been demonstrated inside host cells in the duodenum, but most investigators think this is such an infrequent occurrence that it is not responsible for disease symptoms. Mechanical obstruction of the absorptive surface of the intestine has been proposed as a possible pathogenic mechanism, as has a synergistic relationship with some of the intestinal flora. *Giardia* can be excysted, cultured and encysted in vitro; new isolates have bacterial, fungal, and viral symbionts. Classically the disease was diagnosed by demonstration of the organism in stained fecal smears. Several strains of *G. lamblia* have been isolated and described through analysis of their proteins and DNA; type of strain, however, is not consistently associated with disease severity. Different individuals show various degrees of symptoms when infected with the same strain, and the symptoms of an individual may vary during the course of the disease.

Infectious Dose—Ingestion of one or more cysts may cause disease, as contrasted to most bacterial illnesses where hundreds to thousands of organisms must be consumed to produce illness.

Diagnosis of Human Illness

Giardia lamblia is frequently diagnosed by visualizing the organism, either the trophozoite (active reproducing form) or the cyst (the resting stage that is resistant to adverse environmental conditions) in stained preparations or unstained wet mounts with the aid of a microscope. A commercial fluorescent antibody kit is available to stain the organism. Organisms may be concentrated by sedimentation or flotation; however, these procedures reduce the number of recognizable organisms in the sample. An enzyme linked immunosorbant assay (ELISA) that detects excretory secretory products of the organism is also available. So far, the increased sensitivity of indirect serological detection has not been consistently demonstrated.

Associated Foods

Giardiasis is most frequently associated with the consumption of contaminated water. Five outbreaks have been traced to food contamination by infected or infested food handlers, and the possibility of infections from contaminated vegetables that are eaten raw cannot be excluded. Cool moist conditions favor the survival of the organism.

Relative Frequency of Disease

Giardiasis is more prevalent in children than in adults, possibly because many individuals seem to have a lasting immunity after infection. This organism is implicated in 25% of the cases of gastrointestinal disease and may be present asymptomatically. The overall incidence of infection in the United States is estimated at 2% of the population. This disease afflicts many homosexual men, both HIV-positive and HIV-negative individuals. This is presumed to be due to sexual transmission. The disease is also common in child day care centers, especially those in which diapering is done.

Complications

About 40% of those who are diagnosed with giardiasis demonstrate disaccharide intolerance during detectable infection and up to 6 months after the infection can no longer be detected. Lactose (i.e., milk sugar) intolerance is most frequently observed. Some individuals (less than 4%) remain symptomatic more than 2 weeks; chronic infections lead to a malabsorption syndrome and severe weight loss. Chronic cases of giardiasis in immunodeficient and normal individuals are frequently refractile to drug treatment. Flagyl is normally quite effective in terminating infections. In some immune deficient individuals, giardiasis may contribute to a shortening of the life span.

Target Populations

Giardiasis occurs throughout the population, although the prevalence is higher in children than adults. Chronic symptomatic giardiasis is more common in adults than children.

Food Analysis

Food is analyzed by thorough surface cleaning of the suspected food and sedimentation of the organisms from the cleaning water. Feeding to specific pathogen-free animals has been used to detect the organism in large outbreaks associated with municipal water systems. The precise sensitivity of these methods has not been determined, so that negative results are questionable. Seven days may be required to detect an experimental infection.

Selected Outbreaks

Major outbreaks are associated with contaminated water systems that do not use sand filtration or have a defect in the filtration system. The largest reported foodborne outbreak involved 24 of 36 persons who consumed macaroni salad at a picnic.

For more information on recent outbreaks see the Morbidity and Mortality Weekly Reports from CDC.

FDA Regulations or Activity

FDA is actively developing and improving methods of recovering parasitic protozoa and helminth eggs from foods. Current recovery methods are published in the FDA's Bacteriological Analytical Manual.

Chapter 24

Cryptosporidium

Name of the Organism

Cryptosporidium parvum, a single-celled animal, i.e., a protozoa, is an obligate intracellular parasite. It has been given additional species names when isolated from different hosts. It is currently thought that the form infecting humans is the same species that causes disease in young calves. The forms that infect avian hosts and those that infect mice are not thought capable of infecting humans. *Cryptosporidium* sp. infects many herd animals (cows, goats, sheep among domesticated animals, and deer and elk among wild animals). The infective stage of the organism, the oocyst is 3 um in diameter or about half the size of a red blood cell. The sporocysts are resistant to most chemical disinfectants, but are susceptible to drying and the ultraviolet portion of sunlight. Some strains appear to be adapted to certain hosts but cross-strain infectivity occurs and may or may not be associated with illness. The species or strain infecting the respiratory system is not currently distinguished from the form infecting the intestines.

Disease Name

Intestinal, tracheal, or pulmonary cryptosporidiosis.

Foodborne Pathogenic Microorganisms and Natural Toxins Handbook, January 1992, U.S. Food & Drug Administration, Center for Food Safety & Applied Nutrition.

Nature of Acute Disease

Intestinal cryptosporidiosis is characterized by severe watery diarrhea but may, alternatively, be asymptomatic. Pulmonary and tracheal cryptosporidiosis in humans is associated with coughing and frequently a low-grade fever; these symptoms are often accompanied by severe intestinal distress.

Infectious dose—Less than 10 organisms and, presumably, one organism can initiate an infection. The mechanism of disease is not known; however, the intracellular stages of the parasite can cause severe tissue alteration.

Diagnosis of Human Illness

Oocysts are shed in the infected individual's feces. Sugar flotation is used to concentrate the organisms and acid fast staining is used to identify them. A commercial kit is available that uses fluorescent antibody to stain the organisms isolated from feces. Diagnosis has also been made by staining the trophozoites in intestinal and biopsy specimens. Pulmonary and tracheal cryptosporidiosis are diagnosed by biopsy and staining.

Food Occurrence

Cryptosporidium sp. could occur, theoretically, on any food touched by a contaminated food handler. Incidence is higher in child day care centers that serve food. Fertilizing salad vegetables with manure is another possible source of human infection. Large outbreaks are associated with contaminated water supplies.

Relative Frequency of the Disease

Direct human surveys indicate a prevalence of about 2% of the population in North America. Serological surveys indicate that 80% of the population has had cryptosporidiosis. The extent of illness associated with reactive sera is not known.

Usual Course of the Disease and Complications

Intestinal cryptosporidiosis is self-limiting in most healthy individuals, with watery diarrhea lasting 2-4 days. In some outbreaks at day care centers, diarrhea has lasted 1 to 4 weeks. To date, there is no known effective drug for the treatment of cryptosporidiosis. Immunodeficient individuals, especially AIDS patients, may have the disease for life, with the severe watery diarrhea contributing to death. Invasion of the pulmonary system may also be fatal.

Target Populations

In animals, the young show the most severe symptoms. For the most part, pulmonary infections are confined to those who are immunodeficient. However, an infant with a presumably normal immune system had tracheal cryptosporidiosis (although a concurrent viremia may have accounted for lowered resistance). Child day care centers, with a large susceptible population, frequently report outbreaks.

Analysis of Foods

The 7th edition of FDA's Bacteriological Analytical Manual will contain a method for the examination of vegetables for *Cryptosporidium* sp.

Selected Outbreaks

Since 1984, cryptosporidiosis has been associated with outbreaks of diarrheal illness in child day care centers throughout the United States and Canada. During 1987 a waterborne outbreak in Georgia produced illness in an estimated 13,000 individuals, and exposure to contaminated drinking water was the major distinction between those that were ill and those that were not. This was the first report of disease transmission by a municipal water system that was in compliance with all state and federal standards for drinking water.

An outbreak of cryptosporidiosis associated with the consumption of apple cider is reported in *MMWR* 46(1):1997 Jan 10. *MMWR* 45(36):1996 Sep 13 reports on an outbreak of cryptosporidiosis associated with the consumption of homemade chicken salad in Minnesota.

A non-food outbreak of cryptosporidiosis in a day camp is reported in *MMWR* 45(21):1995 May 31. This report is linked to this chapter to provide reference information.

MMWR 39(20):1990 May 25 reports on a non-food related outbreak of cryptosporidiosis, but contains useful information on *Cryptosporidium* sp.

For more information on recent outbreaks see the *Morbidity and Mortality Weekly Reports* from CDC.

FDA Regulations or Activity

FDA is developing and improving methods for the recovery of cysts of parasitic protozoa from fresh vegetables. Current recovery methods are published in the Bacteriological Analytical Manual.

Education

The CDC has information on *Cryptosporidium.*

Other Resources

From GenBank there is a Loci index for genome *Cryptosporidium parvum.*

Chapter 25

Anisakis Simplex *and Related Worms*

Anisakis simplex (herring worm), *Pseudoterranova (Phocanema, Terranova) decipiens* (cod or seal worm), *Contracaecum spp.*, and *Hysterothylacium (Thynnascaris)* spp. are anisakid nematodes (roundworms) that have been implicated in human infections caused by the consumption of raw or undercooked seafood. To date, only *A. simplex* and *P. decipiens* are reported from human cases in North America.

Name of Acute Disease

Anisakiasis is generally used when referring to the acute disease in humans. Some purists utilize generic names (e.g., contracaeciasis) in referring to the disease, but the majority consider that the name derived from the family is specific enough. The range of clinical features is not dependent on species of anisakid parasite in cases reported to date.

Nature of the Acute Disease

In North America, anisakiasis is most frequently diagnosed when the affected individual feels a tingling or tickling sensation in the throat and coughs up or manually extracts a nematode. In more severe cases there is acute abdominal pain, much like acute appendicitis

Foodborne Pathogenic Microorganisms and Natural Toxins Handbook, January 1992, U.S. Food & Drug Administration, Center for Food Safety & Applied Nutrition.

accompanied by a nauseous feeling. Symptoms occur from as little as an hour to about 2 weeks after consumption of raw or undercooked seafood. One nematode is the usual number recovered from a patient. With their anterior ends, these larval nematodes from fish or shellfish usually burrow into the wall of the digestive tract to the level of the muscularis mucosae (occasionally they penetrate the intestinal wall completely and are found in the body cavity). They produce a substance that attracts eosinophils and other host white blood cells to the area. The infiltrating host cells form a granuloma in the tissues surrounding the penetrated worm. In the digestive tract lumen, the worm can detach and reattach to other sites on the wall. Anisakids rarely reach full maturity in humans and usually are eliminated spontaneously from the digestive tract lumen within 3 weeks of infection. Penetrated worms that die in the tissues are eventually removed by the host's phagocytic cells.

Diagnosis of Human Illness

In cases where the patient vomits or coughs up the worm, the disease may be diagnosed by morphological examination of the nematode. (*Ascaris lumbricoides*, the large roundworm of humans, is a terrestrial relative of anisakines and sometimes these larvae also crawl up into the throat and nasal passages.) Other cases may require a fiber optic device that allows the attending physician to examine the inside of the stomach and the first part of the small intestine. These devices are equipped with a mechanical forceps that can be used to remove the worm. Other cases are diagnosed upon finding a granulomatous lesion with a worm on laparotomy. A specific radioallergosorbent test has been developed for anasakiasis, but is not yet commercially marketed.

Associated Foods

Seafoods are the principal sources of human infections with these larval worms. The adults of *A. simplex* are found in the stomachs of whales and dolphins. Fertilized eggs from the female parasite pass out of the host with the host's feces. In seawater, the eggs embryonate, developing into larvae that hatch in sea water. These larvae are infective to copepods (minute crustaceans related to shrimp) and other small invertebrates. The larvae grow in the invertebrate and become infective for the next host, a fish or larger invertebrate host such as a squid. The larvae may penetrate through the digestive tract into the muscle of the second host. Some evidence exists that the nematode larvae move from the viscera to the flesh if the fish hosts are not gutted promptly after catching. The life cycles of all the other anisakid genera implicated in human infections are similar. These parasites are known to occur frequently in the flesh of cod, haddock, fluke, pacific salmon, herring, flounder, and monkfish.

Relative Frequency of the Disease

Fewer than 10 cases are diagnosed in the U.S. annually. However, it is suspected that many other cases go undetected. The disease is transmitted by raw, undercooked or insufficiently frozen fish and shellfish, and its incidence is expected to increase with the increasing popularity of sushi and sashimi bars.

Usual Disease Course and Complications

Severe cases of anisakiasis are extremely painful and require surgical intervention. Physical removal of the nematode(s) from the lesion is the only known method of reducing the pain and eliminating the cause (other than waiting for the worms to die). The symptoms apparently persist after the worm dies since some lesions are found upon surgical removal that contain only nematode remnants. Stenosis (a narrowing and stiffening) of the pyloric sphincter was reported in a case in which exploratory laparotomy had revealed a worm that was not removed.

Target Populations

The target population consists of consumers of raw or underprocessed seafood.

Analysis of Foods

Candling or examining fish on a light table is used by commercial processors to reduce the number of nematodes in certain white-flesh fish that are known to be infected frequently. This method is not totally effective, nor is it very adequate to remove even the majority of nematodes from fish with pigmented flesh.

Selected Outbreaks

This disease is known primarily from individual cases. Japan has the greatest number of reported cases because of the large volume of raw fish consumed there.

A recent letter to the editor of the *New England Journal of Medicine* (319:1128-29, 1988) stated that approximately 50 cases of anisakiasis have been documented in the United States, to date. Three cases in the San Francisco Bay area involved ingestion of sushi or undercooked fish. The letter also points out that anasakiasis is easily misdiagnosed as acute appendicitis, Crohn's disease, gastric ulcer, or gastrointestinal cancer. For more information on recent outbreaks see the *Morbidity and Mortality Weekly Reports* from CDC.

FDA Activity and Regulations

FDA recommends that all fish and shellfish intended for raw (or semiraw such as marinated or partly cooked) consumption be blast frozen to -35°C (-31°F) or below for 15 hours, or be regularly frozen to -20°C (-4°F) or below for 7 days.

Chapter 26

Acanthamoeba, Naegleria Fowleri *and Other Amobae*

Members of the two genera named above are the principal examples of protozoa commonly referred to as pathogenic free-living amoebae.

Disease Name

Primary amoebic meningoencephalitis (PAM), Naegleria fowleri and granulomatious amoebic encephalitis (GAE), acanthamoebic keratitis or acanthamoebic uveitis.

These organisms are ubiquitous in the environment, in soil, water, and air. Infections in humans are rare and are acquired through water entering the nasal passages (usually during swimming) and by inhalation. They are discussed here because the FDA receives inquiries about them.

Nature of the Acute Disease

PAM occurs in persons who are generally healthy prior to infection. Central nervous system involvement arises from organisms that penetrate the nasal passages and enter the brain through the cribriform plate. The organisms can multiply in the tissues of the central nervous system and may be isolated from spinal fluid. In untreated

Foodborne Pathogenic Microorganisms and Natural Toxins Handbook, January 1992, U.S. Food & Drug Administration, Center for Food Safety & Applied Nutrition.

cases death occurs within 1 week of the onset of symptoms. Amphotercin B is effective in the treatment of PAM. At least four patients have recovered when treated with Amphotercin B alone or in combination with micronazole administered both intravenously and intrathecally or intraventrically.

GAE occurs in persons who are immunodeficient in some way; the organisms cause a granulomatous encephalitis that leads to death in several weeks to a year after the appearance of symptoms. The primary infection site is thought to be the lungs, and the organisms in the brain are generally associated with blood vessels, suggesting vascular dissemination. Treatment with sulfamethazine may be effective in controlling the amobae.

Prior to 1985 amoebae had been reported isolated from diseased eyes only rarely; cases were associated with trauma to the eye. In 1985-1986, 24 eye cases were reported to CDC and most of these occurred in wearers of contact lenses. It has been demonstrated that many of these infections resulted from the use of homemade saline solutions with the contact lenses. Some of the lenses had been heat-treated and others had been chemically disinfected. The failure of the heat treatment was attributed to faulty equipment, since the amoebae are killed by 65°C (149°F) for 30 minutes. The failure of the chemical disinfection resulted from insufficient treatment or rinsing the lenses in contaminated saline after disinfection. The following agents have been used to successfully eliminate the amoebic infection in the eye: ketoconazole, microconazole, and propamidine isothionate; however, penetrating keratoplasty has been necessary to restore useful vision.

Diagnosis of Human Illness

PAM is diagnosed by the presence of amoebae in the spinal fluid. GAE is diagnosed by biopsy of the lesion. Ocular amoebic keratitis may be diagnosed by culturing corneal scrapings on nonnutrient agar overlaid with viable Escherichia coli; amoebae from PAM and GAE may be cultured by the same method. Clinical diagnosis by experienced practitioners is based on the characteristic stromal infiltrate.

Transmission

Transmission is through water-based fluids or the air.

Frequency of Infections

PAM and GAE are rare in occurrence; fewer than 100 cases have been reported in the United States in the 25 years since these diseases were recognized.

Complications

PAM and GAE both lead to death in most cases. Eye infections may lead to blindness.

Target Populations

Immunodeficients, especially those infected with HIV, may be at risk for atypical infections. PAM, GAE, and eye infections have occurred in otherwise healthy individuals.

Food Analysis

Foods are not analyzed for these amoebae since foods are not implicated in the infection of individuals.

Selected Outbreaks

These diseases are known only from isolated cases. For more information on recent outbreaks see the *Morbidity and Mortality Weekly Reports* from CDC.

FDA Activity and Regulations

Since infection is not known to be by way of the digestive tract, the FDA has no regulations concerning these organisms. Eye infections are indirectly regulated by FDA's Center for Medical Devices and Radiological Health; FDA's Center for Drug Evaluation and Research regulates heat sterilization units and saline solutions for ophthalmological use. FDA has published a paper documenting the presence of amoebae in eye wash stations, and warning about the potential danger of such contamination.

Chapter 27

Hepatitis A Virus

Name of the Organism

Hepatitis A virus (HAV) is classified with the enterovirus group of the Picornaviridae family. HAV has a single molecule of RNA surrounded by a small (27 nm diameter) protein capsid and a buoyant density in CsCl of 1.33 g/ml. Many other picornaviruses cause human disease, including polioviruses, coxsackieviruses, echoviruses, and rhinoviruses (cold viruses).

Name of Acute Disease

The term hepatitis A (HA) or type A viral hepatitis has replaced all previous designations: infectious hepatitis, epidemic hepatitis, epidemic jaundice, catarrhal jaundice, infectious icterus, Botkins disease, and MS-1 hepatitis.

Nature of Disease

Hepatitis A is usually a mild illness characterized by sudden onset of fever, malaise, nausea, anorexia, and abdominal discomfort, followed in several days by jaundice. The infectious dose is unknown but presumably is 10-100 virus particles.

Foodborne Pathogenic Microorganisms and Natural Toxins Handbook, January 1992, U.S. Food & Drug Administration, Center for Food Safety & Applied Nutrition.

Diagnosis of Human Illness

Hepatitis A is diagnosed by finding IgM-class anti-HAV in serum collected during the acute or early convalescent phase of disease. Commercial kits are available.

Associated Foods

HAV is excreted in feces of infected people and can produce clinical disease when susceptible individuals consume contaminated water or foods. Cold cuts and sandwiches, fruits and fruit juices, milk and milk products, vegetables, salads, shellfish, and iced drinks are commonly implicated in outbreaks. Water, shellfish, and salads are the most frequent sources. Contamination of foods by infected workers in food processing plants and restaurants is common.

Frequency of Disease

Hepatitis A has a worldwide distribution occurring in both epidemic and sporadic fashions. About 22,700 cases of hepatitis A representing 38% of all hepatitis cases (5-year average from all routes of transmission) are reported annually in the U.S. In 1988 an estimated 7.3% cases were foodborne or waterborne. HAV is primarilly transmitted by person-to-person contact through fecal contamination, but common-source epidemics from contaminated food and water also occur. Poor sanitation and crowding facilitate transmission. Outbreaks of HA are common in institutions, crowded house projects, and prisons and in military forces in adverse situations. In developing countries, the incidence of disease in adults is relatively low because of exposure to the virus in childhood. Most individuals 18 and older demonstrate an immunity that provides lifelong protection against reinfection. In the U.S., the percentage of adults with immunity increases with age (10% for those 18-19 years of age to 65% for those over 50). The increased number of susceptible individuals allows common source epidemics to evolve rapidly.

Usual Course of Disease

The incubation period for hepatitis A, which varies from 10 to 50 days (mean 30 days), is dependent upon the number of infectious particles consumed. Infection with very few particles results in longer incubation periods. The period of communicability extends from early in the incubation period to about a week after the development of jaundice. The greatest danger of spreading the disease to others occurs during the middle of the incubation period, well before the first presentation of symptoms. Many infections with HAV do not result in clinical disease, especially in children. When disease does occur, it is usually mild and recovery is complete in 1-2 weeks. Occasionally, the symptoms are severe and convalescence can take several months. Patients suffer from feeling chronically tired during convalescence, and their inability to work can cause financial loss. Less than 0.4% of the reported cases in the U.S. are fatal. These rare deaths usually occur in the elderly.

Target Population

All people who ingest the virus and are immunologically unprotected are susceptible to infection. Disease however, is more common in adults than in children.

Analysis of Foods

The virus has not been isolated from any food associated with an outbreak. Because of the long incubation period, the suspected food is often no longer available for analysis. No satisfactory method is presently available for routine analysis of food, but sensitive molecular methods used to detect HAV in water and clinical specimens, should prove useful to detect virus in foods. Among those, the PCR amplification method seems particularly promising.

Selected Outbreaks

Hepatitis A is endemic throughout much of the world. Major national epidemics occurred in 1954, 1961 and 1971. Although no major epidemic occurred in the 1980s, the incidence of hepatitis A in the U.S. increased 58% from 1983 to 1989. Foods have been implicated in over 30 outbreaks since 1983. The most recent ones and the suspected contaminated foods include:

- 1987: Louisville, Kentucky—Suspected source: imported lettuce.

- 1988: Alaska—Ice-slush beverage prepared in a local market. North Carolina—Iced tea prepared in a restaurant. Florida— Raw oysters harvested from nonapproved bed.

- 1989: Washington—Unidentified food in a restaurant chain.

- 1990: North Georgia—Frozen strawberries. Montana—Frozen strawberries. Baltimore—Shellfish.

A summary of foodborne Hepatitis A outbreaks in Missouri, Wisconsin, and Alaska is found in *MMWR* 42(27):1993 Jul 16.*MMWR* 39(14):1990 Apr 13 summarizes foodborne outbreaks of Hepatitis A in Alaska, Florida, North Carolina, Washington.

For more information on recent outbreaks see the *Morbidity and Mortality Weekly Reports* from CDC.

Chapter 28

Rotavirus

Name of the Organism

Rotaviruses are classified with the Reoviridae family. They have a genome consisting of 11 double-stranded RNA segments surrounded by a distinctive two-layered protein capsid. Particles are 70 nm in diameter and have a buoyant density of 1.36 g/ml in CsCl. Six serological groups have been identified, three of which (groups A, B, and C) infect humans.

Name of Acute Disease

Rotaviruses cause acute gastroenteritis. Infantile diarrhea, winter diarrhea, acute nonbacterial infectious gastroenteritis, and acute viral gastroenteritis are names applied to the infection caused by the most common and widespread group A rotavirus.

Nature of Disease

Rotavirus gastroenteritis is a self-limiting, mild to severe disease characterized by vomiting, watery diarrhea, and low-grade fever. The infective dose is presumed to be 10-100 infectious viral particles. Because a person with rotavirus diarrhea often excretes large numbers

Foodborne Pathogenic Microorganisms and Natural Toxins Handbook, January 1992, U.S. Food & Drug Administration, Center for Food Safety & Applied Nutrition.

of virus (108-1010 infectious particles/ml of feces), infection doses can be readily acquired through contaminated hands, objects, or utensils. Asymptomatic rotavirus excretion has been well documented and may play a role in perpetuating endemic disease.

Diagnosis of Human Illness

Specific diagnosis of the disease is made by identification of the virus in the patient's stool. Enzyme immunoassay (EIA) is the test most widely used to screen clinical specimens, and several commercial kits are available for group A rotavirus. Electron microscopy (EM) and polyacrylamide gel electrophoresis (PAGE) are used in some laboratories in addition or as an alternative to EIA. A reverse transcription-polymerase chain reaction (RT-PCR) has been developed to detect and identify all three groups of human rotaviruses.

Associated Foods

Rotaviruses are transmitted by the fecal-oral route. Person-to-person spread through contaminated hands is probably the most important means by which rotaviruses are transmitted in close communities such as pediatric and geriatric wards, day care centers and family homes. Infected food handlers may contaminate foods that require handling and no further cooking, such as salads, fruits, and hors d'oeuvres. Rotaviruses are quite stable in the environment and have been found in estuary samples at levels as high as 1-5 infectious particles/gal. Sanitary measures adequate for bacteria and parasites seem to be ineffective in endemic control of rotavirus, as similar incidence of rotavirus infection is observed in countries with both high and low health standards.

Frequency of Disease

Group A rotavirus is endemic worldwide. It is the leading cause of severe diarrhea among infants and children, and accounts for about half of the cases requiring hospitalization. Over 3 million cases of rotavirus gastroenteritis occur annually in the U.S. In temperate areas, it occurs primarily in the winter, but in the tropics it occurs throughout the year. The number attributable to food contamination is unknown.

Group B rotavirus, also called adult diarrhea rotavirus or ADRV, has caused major epidemics of severe diarrhea affecting thousands of persons of all ages in China.

Group C rotavirus has been associated with rare and sporadic cases of diarrhea in children in many countries. However, the first outbreaks were reported from Japan and England.

Usual Course of Disease

The incubation period ranges from 1-3 days. Symptoms often start with vomiting followed by 4-8 days of diarrhea. Temporary lactose intolerance may occur. Recovery is usually complete. However, severe diarrhea without fluid and electrolyte replacement may result in severe diarrhea and death. Childhood mortality caused by rotavirus is relatively low in the U.S., with an estimated 100 cases/year, but reaches almost 1 million cases/year worldwide. Association with other enteric pathogens may play a role in the severity of the disease.

Target Populations

Humans of all ages are susceptible to rotavirus infection. Children 6 months to 2 years of age, premature infants, the elderly, and the immunocompromised are particularly prone to more severe symptoms caused by infection with group A rotavirus.

Analysis of Foods

The virus has not been isolated from any food associated with an outbreak, and no satisfactory method is available for routine analysis of food. However, it should be possible to apply procedures that have been used to detect the virus in water and in clinical specimens, such as enzyme immunoassays, gene probing, and PCR amplification to food analysis.

Selected Outbreaks

Outbreaks of group A rotavirus diarrhea are common among hospitalized infants, young children attending day care centers, and elder persons in nursing homes. Among adults, multiple foods served in banquets were implicated in 2 outbreaks. An outbreak due to contaminated municipal water occurred in Colorado, 1981.

Several large outbreaks of group B rotavirus involving millions of persons as a result of sewage contamination of drinking water supplies have occurred in China since 1982. Although to date outbreaks caused by group B rotavirus have been confined to mainland China, seroepidemiological surveys have indicated lack of immunity to this group of virus in the U.S.

The newly recognized group C rotavirus has been implicated in rare and isolated cases of gastroenteritis. However, it was associated with three outbreaks among school children: one in Japan, 1989, and two in England, 1990.

For a discussion of rotavirus surveillance in the US, see *MMWR* 40(5)1991 Feb 8.

For more information on recent outbreaks see the *Morbidity and Mortality Weekly Reports* from CDC.

Other Resources

From GenBank there is a Loci index for genome Rotavirus sp.

Chapter 29

Various Shellfish-Associated Toxins

Name of Toxins

Shellfish poisoning is caused by a group of toxins elaborated by planktonic algae (dinoflagellates, in most cases) upon which the shellfish feed. The toxins are accumulated and sometimes metabolized by the shellfish. The 20 toxins responsible for paralytic shellfish poisonings (PSP) are all derivatives of saxitoxin. Diarrheic shellfish poisoning (DSP) is presumably caused by a group of high molecular weight polyethers, including okadaic acid, the dinophysis toxins, the pectenotoxins, and yessotoxin. Neurotoxic shellfish poisoning (NSP) is the result of exposure to a group of polyethers called brevetoxins. Amnesic shellfish poisoning (ASP) is caused by the unusual amino acid, domoic acid, as the contaminant of shellfish.

Name of the Acute Diseases

Shellfish Poisoning—Paralytic Shellfish Poisoning (PSP), Diarrheic Shellfish Poisoning (DSP), Neurotoxic Shellfish Poisoning (NSP), Amnesic Shellfish Poisoning (ASP).

Foodborne Pathogenic Microorganisms and Natural Toxins Handbook, January 1992, U.S. Food & Drug Administration, Center for Food Safety & Applied Nutrition.

Nature of the Diseases

Ingestion of contaminated shellfish results in a wide variety of symptoms, depending upon the toxins(s) present, their concentrations in the shellfish and the amount of contaminated shellfish consumed. In the case of PSP, the effects are predominantly neurological and include tingling, burning, numbness, drowsiness, incoherent speech, and respiratory paralysis. Less well characterized are the symptoms associated with DSP, NSP, and ASP. DSP is primarily observed as a generally mild gastrointestinal disorder, i.e., nausea, vomiting, diarrhea, and abdominal pain accompanied by chills, headache, and fever. Both gastrointestinal and neurological symptoms characterize NSP, including tingling and numbness of lips, tongue, and throat, muscular aches, dizziness, reversal of the sensations of hot and cold, diarrhea, and vomiting. ASP is characterized by gastrointestinal disorders (vomiting, diarrhea, abdominal pain) and neurological problems (confusion, memory loss, disorientation, seizure, coma).

Normal Course of the Disease

PSP—Symptoms of the disease develop fairly rapidly, within 0.5 to 2 hours after ingestion of the shellfish, depending on the amount of toxin consumed. In severe cases respiratory paralysis is common, and death may occur if respiratory support is not provided. When such support is applied within 12 hours of exposure, recovery usually is complete, with no lasting side effects. In unusual cases, because of the weak hypotensive action of the toxin, death may occur from cardiovascular collapse despite respiratory support.

NSP—Onset of this disease occurs within a few minutes to a few hours; duration is fairly short, from a few hours to several days. Recovery is complete with few after effects; no fatalities have been reported.

DSP—Onset of the disease, depending on the dose of toxin ingested, may be as little as 30 minutes to 2 to 3 hours, with symptoms of the illness lasting as long as 2 to 3 days. Recovery is complete with no after effects; the disease is generally not life threatening.

ASP—The toxicosis is characterized by the onset of gastrointestinal symptoms within 24 hours; neurological symptoms occur within 48 hours. The toxicosis is particularly serious in elderly patients, and includes symptoms reminiscent of Alzheimer's disease. All fatalities to date have involved elderly patients.

Diagnosis of Human Illnesses

Diagnosis of shellfish poisoning is based entirely on observed symptomatology and recent dietary history.

Associated Foods

All shellfish (filter-feeding molluscs) are potentially toxic. However, PSP is generally associated with mussels, clams, cockles, and scallops; NSP with shellfish harvested along the Florida coast and the Gulf of Mexico; DSP with mussels, oysters, and scallops, and ASP with mussels.

Relative Frequency of Disease

Good statistical data on the occurrence and severity of shellfish poisoning are largely unavailable, which undoubtedly reflects the inability to measure the true incidence of the disease. Cases are frequently misdiagnosed and, in general, infrequently reported. Of these toxicoses, the most serious from a public health perspective appears to be PSP. The extreme potency of the PSP toxins has, in the past, resulted in an unusually high mortality rate.

Target Populations

All humans are susceptible to shellfish poisoning. Elderly people are apparently predisposed to the severe neurological effects of the ASP toxin. A disproportionate number of PSP cases occur among tourists or others who are not native to the location where the toxic shellfish are harvested. This may be due to disregard for either official quarantines or traditions of safe consumption, both of which tend to protect the local population.

Analysis of Foods

The mouse bioassay has historically been the most universally applied technique for examining shellfish (especially for PSP); other bioassay procedures have been developed but not generally applied. Unfortunately, the dose-survival times for the DSP toxins in the mouse assay fluctuate considerably and fatty acids interfere with the assay, giving false-positive results; consequently, a suckling mouse assay that has been developed and used for control of DSP measures fluid accumulation after injection of the shellfish extract. In recent years considerable effort has been applied to development of chemical assays to replace these bioassays. As a result a good high performance liquid chromatography (HPLC) procedure has been developed to identify individual PSP toxins (detection limit for saxitoxin = 20 fg/100 g of meats; 0.2 ppm), an excellent HPLC procedure (detection limit for okadaic acid = 400 ng/g; 0.4 ppm), a commercially available immunoassay (detection limit for okadaic acid = 1 fg/100 g of meats; 0.01 ppm) for DSP and a totally satisfactory HPLC procedure for ASP (detection limit for domoic acid = 750 ng/g; 0.75 ppm).

Selected Outbreaks

PSP is associated with relatively few outbreaks, most likely because of the strong control programs in the United States that prevent human exposure to toxic shellfish. That PSP can be a serious public health problem, however, was demonstrated in Guatemala, where an outbreak of 187 cases with 26 deaths, recorded in 1987, resulted from ingestion of a clam soup. The outbreak led to the establishment of a control program over shellfish harvested in Guatemala.

ASP first came to the attention of public health authorities in 1987 when 156 cases of acute intoxication occurred as a result of ingestion of cultured blue mussels (Mytilus edulis) harvested off Prince Edward Island, in eastern Canada; 22 individuals were hospitalized and three elderly patients eventually died.

The occurrence of DSP in Europe is sporadic, continuous and presumably widespread (anecdotal). DSP poisoning has not been confirmed in U.S. seafood, but the organisms that produce DSP are present in U.S. waters. An outbreak of DSP was recently confirmed in Eastern Canada. Outbreaks of NSP are sporadic and continuous along the Gulf coast of Florida and were recently reported in North Carolina and Texas.

For more information on recent outbreaks see the *Morbidity and Mortality Weekly Reports* from CDC.

Chapter 30

Scombrotoxin

Name of Toxin

Scombrotoxin.

Name of Acute Disease

Scombroid Poisoning (also called Histamine Poisoning). Scombroid poisoning is caused by the ingestion of foods that contain high levels of histamine and possibly other vasoactive amines and compounds. Histamine and other amines are formed by the growth of certain bacteria and the subsequent action of their decarboxylase enzymes on histidine and other amino acids in food, either during the production of a product such as Swiss cheese or by spoilage of foods such as fishery products, particularly tuna or mahi mahi. However, any food that contains the appropriate amino acids and is subjected to certain bacterial contamination and growth may lead to scombroid poisoning when ingested.

Nature of Disease

Initial symptoms may include a tingling or burning sensation in the mouth, a rash on the upper body and a drop in blood pressure.

Foodborne Pathogenic Microorganisms and Natural Toxins Handbook, January 1992, U.S. Food & Drug Administration, Center for Food Safety & Applied Nutrition.

Frequently, headaches and itching of the skin are encountered. The symptoms may progress to nausea, vomiting, and diarrhea and may require hospitalization, particularly in the case of elderly or impaired patients.

Normal Course of Disease

The onset of intoxication symptoms is rapid, ranging from immediate to 30 minutes. The duration of the illness is usually 3 hours, but may last several days.

Diagnosis of Human Illness

Diagnosis of the illness is usually based on the patient's symptoms, time of onset, and the effect of treatment with antihistamine medication. The suspected food must be analyzed within a few hours for elevated levels of histamine to confirm a diagnosis.

Associated Foods

Fishery products that have been implicated in scombroid poisoning include the tunas (e.g., skipjack and yellowfin), mahi mahi, bluefish, sardines, mackerel, amberjack, and abalone. Many other products also have caused the toxic effects. The primary cheese involved in intoxications has been Swiss cheese. The toxin forms in a food when certain bacteria are present and time and temperature permit their growth. Distribution of the toxin within an individual fish fillet or between cans in a case lot can be uneven, with some sections of a product causing illnesses and others not.

Neither cooking, canning, or freezing reduces the toxic effect. Common sensory examination by the consumer cannot ensure the absence or presence of the toxin. Chemical testing is the only reliable test for evaluation of a product.

Relative Frequency of Disease

Scombroid poisoning remains one of the most common forms of fish poisoning in the United States. Even so, incidents of poisoning often go unreported because of the lack of required reporting, a lack of information by some medical personnel, and confusion with the symptoms of other illnesses.

Difficulty with underreporting is a worldwide problem. In the United States from 1968 to 1980, 103 incidents of intoxication involving 827 people were reported. For the same period in Japan, where the quality of fish is a national priority, 42 incidents involving 4,122 people were recorded. Since 1978, 2 actions by FDA have reduced the frequency of intoxications caused by specific products. A defect action level for histamine in canned tuna resulted in increased industry quality control. Secondly, blocklisting of mahi mahi reduced the level of fish imported to the United States.

Target Population

All humans are susceptible to scombroid poisoning; however, the symptoms can be severe for the elderly and for those taking medications such as isoniazid. Because of the worldwide network for harvesting, processing, and distributing fishery products, the impact of the problem is not limited to specific geographical areas of the United States or consumption pattern. These foods are sold for use in homes, schools, hospitals, and restaurants as fresh, frozen, or processed products.

Analysis of Foods

An official method was developed at FDA to determine histamine, using a simple alcoholic extraction and quantitation by fluorescence spectroscopy. There are other untested procedures in the literature.

Selected Outbreaks

Several large outbreaks of scombroid poisoning have been reported. In 1970, some 40 children in a school lunch program became ill from imported canned tuna. In 1973, more than 200 consumers across the United States were affected by domestic canned tuna. In 1979-1980 more than 200 individuals became ill after consuming imported frozen mahi mahi. Symptoms varied with each incident. In the 1973 situation, of the interviewed patients, 86% experienced nausea, 55% diarrhea, 44% headaches and 32% rashes.

Other incidents of intoxication have resulted from the consumption of canned abalone-like products, canned anchovies, and fresh and frozen amberjack, bluefish sole, and scallops. In particular, shipments of unfrozen fish packed in refrigerated containers have posed a significant problem because of inadequate temperature control.

For more information on recent outbreaks see the *Morbidity and Mortality Weekly Reports* from CDC.

Chapter 31

Tetrodotoxin

Name of Toxin

Tetrodotoxin (anhydrotetrodotoxin 4-epitetrodotoxin, tetrodonic acid).

Name of the Acute Disease

Pufferfish Poisoning, Tetradon Poisoning, Fugu Poisoning.

Nature of the Disease

Fish poisoning by consumption of members of the order Tetraodontiformes is one of the most violent intoxications from marine species. The gonads, liver, intestines, and skin of pufferfish can contain levels of tetrodotoxin sufficient to produce rapid and violent death. The flesh of many pufferfish may not usually be dangerously toxic. Tetrodotoxin has also been isolated from widely differing animal species, including the California newt, parrotfish, frogs of the genus Atelopus, the blue-ringed octopus, starfish, angelfish, and xanthid crabs. The metabolic source of tetrodotoxin is uncertain. No algal source has been identified, and until recently tetrodotoxin was assumed to be a metabolic product of the host. However, recent reports of

Foodborne Pathogenic Microorganisms and Natural Toxins Handbook, January 1992, U.S. Food & Drug Administration, Center for Food Safety & Applied Nutrition.

the production of tetrodotoxin/anhydrotetrodotoxin by several bacterial species, including strains of the family Vibrionaceae, Pseudomonas sp., and Photobacterium phosphoreum, point toward a bacterial origin of this family of toxins. These are relatively common marine bacteria that are often associated with marine animals. If confirmed, these findings may have some significance in toxicoses that have been more directly related to these bacterial species.

Normal Course of the Disease

The first symptom of intoxication is a slight numbness of the lips and tongue, appearing between 20 minutes to three hours after eating poisonous pufferfish. The next symptom is increasing paraesthesia in the face and extremities, which may be followed by sensations of lightness or floating. Headache, epigastric pain, nausea, diarrhea, and/or vomiting may occur. Occasionally, some reeling or difficulty in walking may occur. The second stage of the intoxication is increasing paralysis. Many victims are unable to move; even sitting may be difficult. There is increasing respiratory distress. Speech is affected, and the victim usually exhibits dyspnea, cyanosis, and hypotension. Paralysis increases and convulsions, mental impairment, and cardiac arrhythmia may occur. The victim, although completely paralyzed, may be conscious and in some cases completely lucid until shortly before death. Death usually occurs within 4 to 6 hours, with a known range of about 20 minutes to 8 hours.

Diagnosis of Human Illness

The diagnosis of pufferfish poisoning is based on the observed symptomology and recent dietary history.

Associated Foods

Poisonings from tetrodotoxin have been almost exclusively associated with the consumption of pufferfish from waters of the Indo-Pacific ocean regions. Several reported cases of poisonings, including fatalities, involved pufferfish from the Atlantic Ocean, Gulf of Mexico, and Gulf of California. There have been no confirmed cases of poisoning from the Atlantic pufferfish, Spheroides maculatus. However, in one study, extracts from fish of this species were highly toxic in mice. The trumpet shell Charonia sauliae has been implicated in food poisonings, and evidence suggests that it contains a tetrodotoxin derivative.

There have been several reported poisonings from mislabeled pufferfish and at least one report of a fatal episode when an individual swallowed a California newt.

Relative Frequency of Disease

From 1974 through 1983 there were 646 reported cases of pufferfish poisoning in Japan, with 179 fatalities. Estimates as high as 200 cases per year with mortality approaching 50% have been reported. Only a few cases have been reported in the United States, and outbreaks in countries outside the Indo-Pacific area are rare.

Target Population

All humans are susceptible to tetrodotoxin poisoning. This toxicosis may be avoided by not consuming pufferfish or other animal species containing tetrodotoxin. Most other animal species known to contain tetrodotoxin are not usually consumed by humans. Poisoning from tetrodotoxin is of major public health concern primarily in Japan, where "fugu" is a traditional delicacy. It is prepared and sold in special restaurants where trained and licensed individuals carefully remove the viscera to reduce the danger of poisoning. Importation of pufferfish into the United States is not generally permitted, although special exceptions may be granted. There is potential for misidentification and/or mislabeling, particularly of prepared, frozen fish products.

Analysis of Foods

The mouse bioassay developed for paralytic shellfish poisoning (PSP) can be used to monitor tetrodotoxin in pufferfish and is the current method of choice. An HPLC method with post-column reaction with alkali and fluorescence has been developed to determine tetrodotoxin and its associated toxins. The alkali degradation products can be confirmed as their trimethylsilyl derivatives by gas chromatography/mass spectrometry. These chromatographic methods have not yet been validated.

Selected Outbreaks

Pufferfish poisoning is a continuing problem in Japan, affecting 30-100 persons/year. Most of these poisoning episodes occur from home preparation and consumption and not from commercial sources of the pufferfish. Three deaths were reported in Italy in 1977 following the consumption of frozen pufferfish imported from Taiwan and mis-labeled as angler fish.

An incident of Fugu fish poisoning in the United States is reported in MMWR 45(19):1996 May 17.

For more information on recent outbreaks see the *Morbidity and Mortality Weekly Reports* from CDC.

Chapter 32

Mushroom Toxins

Name of Toxin(s)

Amanitin, Gyromitrin, Orellanine, Muscarine, Ibotenic Acid, Muscimol, Psilocybin, Coprine.

Name of Acute Disease

Mushroom Poisoning, Toadstool Poisoning.

Mushroom poisoning is caused by the consumption of raw or cooked fruiting bodies (mushrooms, toadstools) of a number of species of higher fungi. The term toadstool (from the German Todesstuhl, death's stool) is commonly given to poisonous mushrooms, but for individuals who are not experts in mushroom identification there are generally no easily recognizable differences between poisonous and nonpoisonous species. Old wives' tales notwithstanding, there is no general rule of thumb for distinguishing edible mushrooms and poisonous toadstools. The toxins involved in mushroom poisoning are produced naturally by the fungi themselves, and each individual specimen of a toxic species should be considered equally poisonous. Most mushrooms that cause human poisoning cannot be made nontoxic by cooking, canning, freezing, or any other means of processing. Thus, the only way to avoid poisoning is to avoid consumption of the toxic

Foodborne Pathogenic Microorganisms and Natural Toxins Handbook, January 1992, U.S. Food & Drug Administration, Center for Food Safety & Applied Nutrition.

species. Poisonings in the United States occur most commonly when hunters of wild mushrooms (especially novices) misidentify and consume a toxic species, when recent immigrants collect and consume a poisonous American species that closely resembles an edible wild mushroom from their native land, or when mushrooms that contain psychoactive compounds are intentionally consumed by persons who desire these effects.

Nature of Disease(s)

Mushroom poisonings are generally acute and are manifested by a variety of symptoms and prognoses, depending on the amount and species consumed. Because the chemistry of many of the mushroom toxins (especially the less deadly ones) is still unknown and positive identification of the mushrooms is often difficult or impossible, mushroom poisonings are generally categorized by their physiological effects. There are four categories of mushroom toxins: protoplasmic poisons (poisons that result in generalized destruction of cells, followed by organ failure); neurotoxins (compounds that cause neurological symptoms such as profuse sweating, coma, convulsions, hallucinations, excitement, depression, spastic colon); gastrointestinal irritants (compounds that produce rapid, transient nausea, vomiting, abdominal cramping, and diarrhea); and disulfiram-like toxins. Mushrooms in this last category are generally nontoxic and produce no symptoms unless alcohol is consumed within 72 hours after eating them, in which case a short-lived acute toxic syndrome is produced.

Normal Course of Disease(s)

The normal course of the disease varies with the dose and the mushroom species eaten. Each poisonous species contains one or more toxic compounds which are unique to few other species. Therefore, cases of mushroom poisonings generally do not resembles each other unless they are caused by the same or very closely related mushroom species. Almost all mushroom poisonings may be grouped in one of the categories outlined above.

Protoplasmic Poisons

Amatoxins: Several mushroom species, including the Death Cap or Destroying Angel (*Amanita phalloides, A. virosa*), the Fool's Mushroom (*A. verna*) and several of their relatives, along with the Autumn

Skullcap (*Galerina autumnalis*) and some of its relatives, produce a family of cyclic octapeptides called amanitins. Poisoning by the amanitins is characterized by a long latent period (range 6-48 hours, average 6-15 hours) during which the patient shows no symptoms. Symptoms appear at the end of the latent period in the form of sudden, severe seizures of abdominal pain, persistent vomiting and watery diarrhea, extreme thirst, and lack of urine production. If this early phase is survived, the patient may appear to recover for a short time, but this period will generally be followed by a rapid and severe loss of strength, prostration, and pain-caused restlessness. Death in 50-90% of the cases from progressive and irreversible liver, kidney, cardiac, and skeletal muscle damage may follow within 48 hours (large dose), but the disease more typically lasts 6 to 8 days in adults and 4 to 6 days in children. Two or three days after the onset of the later phase, jaundice, cyanosis, and coldness of the skin occur. Death usually follows a period of coma and occasionally convulsions. If recovery occurs, it generally requires at least a month and is accompanied by enlargement of the liver. Autopsy will usually reveal fatty degeneration and necrosis of the liver and kidney.

Hydrazines: Certain species of False Morel (*Gyromitra esculenta* and *G. gigas*) contain the protoplasmic poison gyromitrin, a volatile hydrazine derivative. Poisoning by this toxin superficially resembles Amanita poisoning but is less severe. There is generally a latent period of 6-10 hours after ingestion during which no symptoms are evident, followed by sudden onset of abdominal discomfort (a feeling of fullness), severe headache, vomiting, and sometimes diarrhea. The toxin affects primarily the liver, but there are additional disturbances to blood cells and the central nervous system. The mortality rate is relatively low (2-4%). Poisonings with symptoms almost identical to those produced by Gyromitra have also been reported after ingestion of the Early False Morel (*Verpa bohemica*). The toxin is presumed to be related to gyromitrin but has not yet been identified.

Orellanine: The final type of protoplasmic poisoning is caused by the Sorrel Webcap mushroom (*Cortinarius orellanus*) and some of its relatives. This mushroom produces orellanine, which causes a type of poisoning characterized by an extremely long asymptomatic latent period of 3 to 14 days. An intense, burning thirst (polydipsia) and excessive urination (polyuria) are the first symptoms. This may be followed by nausea, headache, muscular pains, chills, spasms, and loss of consciousness. In severe cases, severe renal tubular necrosis and kidney failure may result in death (15%) several weeks after the poisoning. Fatty degeneration of the liver and severe inflammatory changes in the intestine accompany the renal damage, and recovery in less severe cases may require several months.

Neurotoxins

Poisonings by mushrooms that cause neurological problems may be divided into three groups, based on the type of symptoms produced, and named for the substances responsible for these symptoms.

Muscarine Poisoning: Ingestion of any number of Inocybe or Clitocybe species (e.g., *Inocybe geophylla, Clitocybe* dealbata) results in an illness characterized primarily by profuse sweating. This effect is caused by the presence in these mushrooms of high levels (3-4%) of muscarine. Muscarine poisoning is characterized by increased salivation, perspiration, and lacrimation within 15 to 30 minutes after ingestion of the mushroom. With large doses, these symptoms may be followed by abdominal pain, severe nausea, diarrhea, blurred vision, and labored breathing. Intoxication generally subsides within 2 hours. Deaths are rare, but may result from cardiac or respiratory failure in severe cases.

Ibotenic acid/Muscimol Poisoning: The Fly Agaric (*Amanita muscaria*) and Panthercap (*Amanita pantherina*) mushrooms both produce ibotenic acid and muscimol. Both substances produce the same effects, but muscimol is approximately 5 times more potent than ibotenic acid. Symptoms of poisoning generally occur within 1- 2 hours after ingestion of the mushrooms. An initial abdominal discomfort may be present or absent, but the chief symptoms are drowsiness and dizziness (sometimes accompanied by sleep), followed by a period of hyperactivity, excitability, illusions, and delirium. Periods of drowsiness may alternate with periods of excitement, but symptoms generally fade within a few hours. Fatalities rarely occur in adults, but in children, accidental consumption of large quantities of these mushrooms may cause convulsions, coma, and other neurologic problems for up to 12 hours.

Psilocybin Poisoning: A number of mushrooms belonging to the genera *Psilocybe, Panaeolus, Copelandia, Gymnopilus, Conocybe,* and *Pluteus,* when ingested, produce a syndrome similar to alcohol intoxication (sometimes accompanied by hallucinations). Several of these mushrooms (e.g., *Psilocybe cubensis*, *P. mexicana*, *Conocybe cyanopus*) are eaten for their psychotropic effects in religious ceremonies of certain native American tribes, a practice which dates to the pre-Columbian era. The toxic effects are caused by psilocin and psilocybin. Onset of symptoms is usually rapid and the effects generally subside within 2 hours. Poisonings by these mushrooms are rarely fatal in adults and may be distinguished from ibotenic acid poisoning by the absence of drowsiness or coma. The most severe cases of psilocybin poisoning occur in small children, where large doses may cause the hallucinations accompanied by fever, convulsions, coma, and death. These mushrooms are generally small, brown, nondescript, and not particularly fleshy; they are seldom mistaken for food fungi by innocent hunters of wild mushrooms. Poisonings caused by intentional ingestion of these mushrooms by people with no legitimate religious justification must be handled with care, since the only cases likely to be seen by the physician are overdoses or intoxications caused by a combination of the mushroom and some added psychotropic substance (such as PCP).

Gastrointestinal Irritants

Numerous mushrooms, including the Green Gill (*Chlorophyllum molybdites*), Gray Pinkgill (*Entoloma lividum*), Tigertop (*Tricholoma pardinum*), Jack O'Lantern (*Omphalotus illudens*), Naked Brimcap (*Paxillus involutus*), Sickener (*Russula emetica*), Early False Morel (*Verpa bohemica*), Horse mushroom (*Agaricus arvensis*) and Pepper bolete (*Boletus piperatus*), contain toxins that can cause gastrointestinal distress, including but not limited to nausea, vomiting, diarrhea, and abdominal cramps. In many ways these symptoms are similar to those caused by the deadly protoplasmic poisons. The chief and diagnostic difference is that poisonings caused by these mushrooms have a rapid onset, rather than the delayed onset seen in protoplasmic poisonings. Some mushrooms (including the first five species mentioned above) may cause vomiting and/or diarrhea which lasts for several days. Fatalities caused by these mushrooms are relatively rare and are associated with dehydration and electrolyte imbalances caused by diarrhea and vomiting, especially in debilitated, very young, or very old patients. Replacement of fluids and other appropriate supportive therapy will prevent death in these cases. The chemistry of the toxins responsible for this type of poisoning is virtually unknown, but may be related to the presence in some mushrooms of unusual sugars, amino acids, peptides, resins, and other compounds.

Disulfiram-Like Poisoning

The Inky Cap Mushroom (*Coprinus atramentarius*) is most commonly responsible for this poisoning, although a few other species have also been implicated. A complicating factor in this type of intoxication is that this species is generally considered edible (i.e., no illness results when eaten in the absence of alcoholic beverages). The mushroom produces an unusual amino acid, coprine, which is converted to cyclopropanone hydrate in the human body. This compound interferes with the breakdown of alcohol, and consumption of alcoholic beverages within 72 hours after eating it will cause headache, nausea and vomiting, flushing, and cardiovascular disturbances that last for 2 - 3 hours.

Miscellaneous Poisonings

Young fruiting bodies of the sulfur shelf fungus Laetiporus sulphureus are considered edible. However, ingestion of this shelf fungus has caused digestive upset and other symptoms in adults and visual hallucinations and ataxia in a child.

Diagnosis of Human Illness

A clinical testing procedure is currently available only for the most serious types of mushroom toxins, the amanitins. The commercially available method uses a 3H-radioimmunoassay (RIA) test kit and can detect sub-nanogram levels of toxin in urine and plasma. Unfortunately, it requires a 2-hour incubation period, and this is an excruciating delay in a type of poisoning which the clinician generally does not see until a day or two has passed. A 125I-based kit which overcomes this problem has recently been reported, but has not yet reached the clinic. A sensitive and rapid HPLC technique has been reported in the literature even more recently, but it has not yet seen clinical application. Since most clinical laboratories in this country do not use even the older RIA technique, diagnosis is based entirely on symptomology and recent dietary history. Despite the fact that cases of mushroom poisoning may be broken down into a relatively small number of categories based on symptomatology, positive botanical identification of the mushroom species consumed remains the only means of unequivocally determining the particular type of intoxication involved, and it is still vitally important to obtain such accurate identification as quickly as possible. Cases involving ingestion of more than one toxic species in which one set of symptoms masks or mimics another set are among many reasons for needing this information. Unfortunately, a number of factors (not discussed here) often make identification of the causative mushroom impossible. In such cases, diagnosis must be based on symptoms alone. In order to rule out other types of food poisoning and to conclude that the mushrooms eaten were the cause of the poisoning, it must be established that everyone who ate the suspect mushrooms became ill and that no one who did not eat the mushrooms became ill. Wild mushrooms eaten raw, cooked, or processed should always be regarded as prime suspects. After ruling out other sources of food poisoning and positively implicating mushrooms as the cause of the illness, diagnosis may proceed in two steps. The first step provides an early indication of the seriousness of the disease and its prognosis.

As described above, the protoplasmic poisons are the most likely to be fatal or to cause irreversible organ damage. In the case of poisoning by the deadly Amanitas, important laboratory indicators of liver (elevated LDH, SGOT, and bilirubin levels) and kidney (elevated uric acid, creatinine, and BUN levels) damage will be present. Unfortunately, in the absence of dietary history, these signs could be mistaken for symptoms of liver or kidney impairment as the result of other causes (e.g., viral hepatitis). It is important that this distinction be made as quickly as possible, because the delayed onset of symptoms will generally mean that the organ has already been damaged. The importance of rapid diagnosis is obvious: victims who are hospitalized and given aggressive support therapy almost immediately after ingestion have a mortality rate of only 10%, whereas those admitted 60 or more hours after ingestion have a 50-90% mortality rate. A recent report indicates that amanitins are observable in urine well before the onset of any symptoms, but that laboratory tests for liver dysfunction do not appear until well after the organ has been damaged.

Associated Foods

Mushroom poisonings are almost always caused by ingestion of wild mushrooms that have been collected by nonspecialists (although specialists have also been poisoned). Most cases occur when toxic species are confused with edible species, and a useful question to ask of the victims or their mushroom-picking benefactors is the identity of the mushroom they thought they were picking. In the absence of a well-preserved specimen, the answer to this question could narrow the possible suspects considerably. Intoxication has also occurred when reliance was placed on some folk method of distinguishing poisonous and safe species. Outbreaks have occurred after ingestion of fresh, raw mushrooms, stir-fried mushrooms, home-canned mushrooms, mushrooms cooked in tomato sauce (which rendered the sauce itself toxic, even when no mushrooms were consumed), and mushrooms that were blanched and frozen at home. Cases of poisoning by home-canned and frozen mushrooms are especially insidious because a single outbreak may easily become a multiple outbreak when the preserved toadstools are carried to another location and consumed at another time.

Specific cases of mistaken mushroom identity appears frequently. The Early False Morel Gyromitra esculenta is easily confused with the true Morel *Morchella esculenta*, and poisonings have occurred after consumption of fresh or cooked Gyromitra. Gyromitra poisonings have also occurred after ingestion of commercially available "morels" contaminated with *G. esculenta*. The commercial sources for these fungi (which have not yet been successfully cultivated on a large scale) are field collection of wild morels by semiprofessionals. Cultivated commercial mushrooms of whatever species are almost never implicated in poisoning outbreaks unless there are associated problems such as improper canning (which lead to bacterial food poisoning). Producers of mild gastroenteritis are too numerous to list here, but include members of many of the most abundant genera, including *Agaricus, Boletus, Lactarius, Russula, Tricholoma, Coprinus, Pluteus,* and others. The Inky Cap Mushroom (*Coprinus atrimentarius*) is considered both edible and delicious, and only the unwary who consume alcohol after eating this mushroom need be concerned. Some other members of the genus *Coprinus* (Shaggy Mane, *C. comatus*; Glistening Inky Cap, *C. micaceus,* and others) and some of the larger members of the Lepiota family such as the Parasol Mushroom (*Leucocoprinus procera*) do not contain coprine and do not cause this effect. The potentially deadly Sorrel Webcap Mushroom (*Cortinarius orellanus*) is not easily distinguished from nonpoisonous webcaps belonging to the same distinctive genus, and all should be avoided.

Most of the psychotropic mushrooms (*Inocybe* spp., *Conocybe* spp., *Paneolus* spp., *Pluteus* spp.) are in general appearance small, brown, and leathery (the so-called "Little Brown Mushrooms" or LBMs) and relatively unattractive from a culinary standpoint. The Sweat Mushroom (*Clitocybe* dealbata) and the Smoothcap Mushroom (*Psilocybe cubensis*) are small, white, and leathery. These small, unattractive mushrooms are distinctive, fairly unappetizing, and not easily confused with the fleshier fungi normally considered edible. Intoxications associated with them are less likely to be accidental, although both *C. dealbata* and *Paneolus foenisicii* have been found growing in the same fairy ring area as the edible (and choice) Fairy Ring Mushroom (*Marasmius oreades*) and the Honey Mushroom (*Armillariella mellea*), and have been consumed when the picker has not carefully examined every mushroom picked from the ring. Psychotropic mushrooms, which are larger and therefore more easily confused with edible mushrooms, include the Showy Flamecap or Big Laughing Mushroom (*Gymnopilus spectabilis*), which has been mistaken for Chanterelles (*Cantharellus* spp.) and for *Gymnopilus* ventricosus found growing on wood of conifers in western North America. The Fly Agaric (*Amanita muscaria*) and Panthercap (*Amanita pantherina*) mushrooms are large, fleshy, and colorful. Yellowish cap colors on some varieties of the Fly Agaric and the Panthercap are similar to the edible Caesar's Mushroom (*Amanita caesarea*), which is considered a delicacy in Italy. Another edible yellow capped mushroom occasionally confused with yellow A. muscaria and A. pantherina varieties are the Yellow Blusher (*Amanita flavorubens*). Orange to yellow-orange A. muscaria and A. pantherina may also be confused with the Blusher (*Amanita rubescens*) and the Honey Mushroom (*Armillariella mellea*). White to pale forms of A. muscaria may be confused with edible field mushrooms (*Agaricus* spp.). Young (button stage) specimens of *A. muscaria* have also been confused with puffballs.

Relative Frequency of Disease

Accurate figures on the relative frequency of mushroom poisonings are difficult to obtain. For the 5-year period between 1976 and 1981, 16 outbreaks involving 44 cases were reported to the Centers for Disease Control in Atlanta (Rattanvilay et al. *MMWR* 31(21): 287-288, 1982). The number of unreported cases is, of course, unknown. Cases are sporadic and large outbreaks are rare. Poisonings tend to be grouped in the spring and fall when most mushroom species are at the height of their fruiting stage. While the actual incidence appears to be very low, the potential exists for grave problems. Poisonous mushrooms are not limited in distribution as are other poisonous organisms (such as dinoflagellates). Intoxications may occur at any time and place, with dangerous species occurring in habitats ranging from urban lawns to deep woods. As Americans become more adventurous in their mushroom collection and consumption, poisonings are likely to increase.

Target Population

All humans are susceptible to mushroom toxins. The poisonous species are ubiquitous, and geographical restrictions on types of poisoning that may occur in one location do not exist (except for some of the hallucinogenic LBMs, which occur primarily in the American southwest and southeast). Individual specimens of poisonous mushrooms are also characterized by individual variations in toxin content based on genetics, geographic location, and growing conditions. Intoxications may thus be more or less serious, depending not on the number of mushrooms consumed, but on the dose of toxin delivered. In addition, although most cases of poisoning by higher plants occur in children, toxic mushrooms are consumed most often by adults. Occasional accidental mushroom poisonings of children and pets have been reported, but adults are more likely to actively search for and consume wild mushrooms for culinary purposes. Children are more seriously affected by the normally nonlethal toxins than are adults and are more likely to suffer very serious consequences from ingestion of relatively smaller doses. Adults who consume mushrooms are also more likely to recall what was eaten and when, and are able to describe their symptoms more accurately than are children. Very old, very young, and debilitated persons of both sexes are more likely to become seriously ill from all types of mushroom poisoning, even those types which are generally considered to be mild.

Many idiosyncratic adverse reactions to mushrooms have been reported. Some mushrooms cause certain people to become violently ill, while not affecting others who consumed part of the same mushroom cap. Factors such as age, sex, and general health of the consumer do not seem to be reliable predictors of these reactions, and they have been attributed to allergic or hypersensitivity reactions and to inherited inability of the unfortunate victim to metabolize certain unusual fungal constituents (such as the uncommon sugar, trehalose). These reactions are probably not true poisonings as the general population does not seem to be affected.

Analysis of Foods for Toxins

The mushroom toxins can with difficulty be recovered from poisonous fungi, cooking water, stomach contents, serum, and urine. Procedures for extraction and quantitation are generally elaborate and time-consuming, and the patient will in most cases have recovered by the time an analysis is made on the basis of toxin chemistry. The exact chemical natures of most of the toxins that produce milder symptoms are unknown. Chromatographic techniques (TLC, GLC, HPLC) exist for the amanitins, orellanine, muscimol/ibotenic acid, psilocybin, muscarine, and the gyromitrins. The amanitins may also be determined by commercially available 3H-RIA kits. The most reliable means of diagnosing a mushroom poisoning remains botanical identification of the fungus that was eaten. An accurate pre-ingestion determination of species will also prevent accidental poisoning in 100% of cases. Accurate post-ingestion analyses for specific toxins when no botanical identification is possible may be essential only in cases of suspected poisoning by the deadly Amanitas, since prompt and aggressive therapy (including lavage, activated charcoal, and plasmapheresis) can greatly reduce the mortality rate.

Selected Outbreaks

Isolated cases of mushroom poisoning have occurred throughout the continental United States. The occurred in Oregon in October, 1988, and involved the intoxication of five people who consumed stir-fried Amanita phalloides. The poisonings were severe, and at this writing three of the five people had undergone liver transplants for treatment of amanitin-induced liver failure. Other recent cases have included the July, 1986, poisoning of a family in Philadelphia, by Chlorophyllum molybdites; the September, 1987, intoxication of seven men in Bucks County, PA, by spaghetti sauce which contained Jack O'Lantern mushroom (*Omphalotus illudens*); and of 14 teenage campers in Maryland by the same species (July, 1987). A report of a North Carolina outbreak of poisoning by False Morel (*Gyromitra* spp.) appeared in 1986. A 1985 report details a case of *Chlorophyllum molybdites* which occurred in Arkansas; a fatal poisoning case caused by an amanitin containing Lepiota was described in 1986. In 1981, two Berks County, PA, people were poisoned (one fatally) after ingesting Amanita phalloides, while in the same year, seven Laotian refugees living in California were poisoned by Russula spp. In separate 1981 incidents, several people from New York State were poisoned by Omphalotus illudens, Amanita muscaria, Entoloma lividum, and Amanita virosa. An outbreak of gastroenteritis during a banquet for 482 people in Vancouver, British Columbia, was reported by the Vancouver Health Department in June, 1991. Seventy-seven of the guests reported symptoms consisting of early onset nausea (15-30 min), diarrhea (20 min-13 h), vomiting (20-60 min), cramps and bloated feeling. Other symptoms included feeling warm, clamminess, numbness of the tongue and extreme thirst along with two cases of hive-like rash with onset of 3-7 days. Bacteriological tests were negative. This intoxication merits special attention because it involved consumption of species normally considered not only edible but choice. The fungi involved were the morels *Morchella esculenta* and *M. elata* (*M. angusticeps*), which were prepared in a marinade and consumed raw. The symptoms were severe but not life threatening. Scattered reports of intoxications by these species and *M. conica* have appeared in anecodotal reports for many years.

Numerous other cases exist; however, the cases that appear in the literature tend to be the serious poisonings such as those causing more severe gastrointestinal symptoms, psychotropic reactions, and severe organ damage (deadly Amanita). Mild intoxications are probably grossly underreported, because of the lack of severity of symptoms and the unlikeliness of a hospital admission.

For more information on recent outbreaks see the *Morbidity and Mortality Weekly Reports* from CDC.

Chapter 33

Phytohaemagglutinin

Name of the Toxin

Phytohaemagglutinin (Kidney Bean Lectin). This compound, a lectin or hemagglutinin, has been used by immunologists for years to trigger DNA synthesis in T lymphocytes, and more recently, to activate latent human immunodeficiency virus type 1 (HIV-1, AIDS virus) from human peripheral lymphocytes. Besides inducing mitosis, lectins are known for their ability to agglutinate many mammalian red blood cell types, alter cell membrane transport systems, alter cell permeability to proteins, and generally interfere with cellular metabolism.

Name of the Acute Disease

Red Kidney Bean (*Phaseolus vulgaris*) Poisoning, Kinkoti Bean Poisoning, and possibly other names.

Nature of the Acute Disease

The onset time from consumption of raw or undercooked kidney beans to symptoms varies from between 1 to 3 hours. Onset is usually marked by extreme nausea, followed by vomiting, which may be very severe. Diarrhea develops somewhat later (from one to a few

Foodborne Pathogenic Microorganisms and Natural Toxins Handbook, January 1992, U.S. Food & Drug Administration, Center for Food Safety & Applied Nutrition.

hours), and some persons report abdominal pain. Some persons have been hospitalized, but recovery is usually rapid (3 - 4 hours after on-set of symptoms) and spontaneous.

Diagnosis of Human Illness

Diagnosis is made on the basis of symptoms, food history, and the exclusion of other rapid onset food poisoning agents (e.g., *Bacillus cereus*, *Staphylococcus aureus*, arsenic, mercury, lead, and cyanide).

Foods in Which It Occurs

Phytohaemagglutinin, the presumed toxic agent, is found in many species of beans, but it is in highest concentration in red kidney beans (*Phaseolus vulgaris*). The unit of toxin measure is the hemagglutinating unit (hau). Raw kidney beans contain from 20,000 to 70,000 hau, while fully cooked beans contain from 200 to 400 hau. White kidney beans, another variety of *Phaseolus vulgaris*, contain about one-third the amount of toxin as the red variety; broad beans (*Vicia faba*) contain 5 to 10% the amount that red kidney beans contain.

The syndrome is usually caused by the ingestion of raw, soaked kidney beans, either alone or in salads or casseroles. As few as four or five raw beans can trigger symptoms. Several outbreaks have been associated with "slow cookers" or crock pots, or in casseroles which had not reached a high enough internal temperature to destroy the glycoprotein lectin. It has been shown that heating to 80°C may potentiate the toxicity five-fold, so that these beans are more toxic than if eaten raw. In studies of casseroles cooked in slow cookers, internal temperatures often did not exceed 75°C.

Frequency of the Disease

This syndrome has occurred in the United Kingdom with some regularity. Seven outbreaks occurred in the U.K. between 1976 and 1979 and were reviewed (Noah et al. 1980. *Br. Med. J.* 19 July, 236-7). Two more incidents were reported by Public Health Laboratory Services (PHLS), Colindale, U.K. in the summer of 1988. Reports of this syndrome in the United States are anecdotal and have not been formally published.

Usual Course of the Disease and Some Complications

The disease course is rapid. All symptoms usually resolve within several hours of onset. Vomiting is usually described as profuse, and the severity of symptoms is directly related to the dose of toxin (number of raw beans ingested). Hospitalization has occasionally resulted, and intravenous fluids may have to be administered. Although of short duration, the symptoms are extremely debilitating.

Target Populations

All persons, regardless of age or gender, appear to be equally susceptible; the severity is related only to the dose ingested. In the seven outbreaks mentioned above, the attack rate was 100%.

Analysis of Food

The difficulty in food analysis is that this syndrome is not well known in the medical community. Other possible causes must be eliminated, such as *Bacillus cereus*, *staphylococcal* food poisoning, or chemical toxicity. If beans are a component of the suspected meal, analysis is quite simple, and based on hemagglutination of red blood cells (hau).

Selected Outbreaks

As previously stated, no major outbreaks have occurred in the U.S. Outbreaks in the U.K. are far more common. The syndrome is probably sporadic, affecting small numbers of persons or individuals, and is easily misdiagnosed or never reported due to the short duration of symptoms. Differences in reporting between the U.S. and U.K. may be attributed to greater use of dried kidney beans in the U.K., or better physician awareness. The U.K. has established a reference laboratory for the quantitation of hemagglutinins from suspected foods.

For more information on recent outbreaks see the *Morbidity and Mortality Weekly Reports* from CDC.

Education

NOTE: The following procedure has been recommended by the PHLS to render kidney, and other, beans safe for consumption:

- Soak in water for at least 5 hours.
- Pour away the water.
- Boil briskly in fresh water for at least 10 minutes.
- Undercooked beans may be more toxic than raw beans.

Chapter 34

Grayanotoxin

Name of Toxin

Grayanotoxin (formerly known as andromedotoxin, acetylandromedol, and rhodotoxin).

Name of Acute Disease

Honey intoxication is caused by the consumption of honey produced from the nectar of rhododendrons. The grayanotoxins cause the intoxication. The specific grayanotoxins vary with the plant species. These compounds are diterpenes, polyhydroxylated cyclic hydrocarbons that do not contain nitrogen. Other names associated with the disease is rhododendron poisoning, mad honey intoxication or grayanotoxin poisoning.

Nature of Disease

The intoxication is rarely fatal and generally lasts for no more than 24 hours. Generally the disease induces dizziness, weakness, excessive perspiration, nausea, and vomiting shortly after the toxic honey is ingested. Other symptoms that can occur are low blood pressure or shock, bradyarrhythima (slowness of the heart beat associated with

Foodborne Pathogenic Microorganisms and Natural Toxins Handbook, January 1992, U.S. Food & Drug Administration, Center for Food Safety & Applied Nutrition.

an irregularity in the heart rhythm), sinus bradycardia (a slow sinus rhythm, with a heart rate less than 60), nodal rhythm (pertaining to a node, particularly the atrioventricular node), Wolff-Parkinson-White syndrome (anomalous atrioventricular excitation) and complete atrioventricular block.

Normal Course of the Disease

The grayanotoxins bind to sodium channels in cell membranes. The binding unit is the group II receptor site, localized on a region of the sodium channel that is involved in the voltage-dependent activation and inactivation. These compounds prevent inactivation; thus, excitable cells (nerve and muscle) are maintained in a state of depolarization, during which entry of calcium into the cells may be facilitated. This action is similar to that exerted by the alkaloids of veratrum and aconite. All of the observed responses of skeletal and heart muscles, nerves, and the central nervous system are related to the membrane effects.

Because the intoxication is rarely fatal and recovery generally occurs within 24 hours, intervention may not be required. Severe low blood pressure usually responds to the administration of fluids and correction of bradycardia; therapy with vasopressors (agents that stimulate contraction of the muscular tissue of the capillaries and arteries) is only rarely required. Sinus bradycardia and conduction defects usually respond to atropine therapy; however, in at least one instance the use of a temporary pacemaker was required.

Diagnosis of Human Illness

In humans, symptoms of poisoning occur after a dose-dependent latent period of a few minutes to two or more hours and include salivation, vomiting, and both circumoral (around or near the mouth) and extremity paresthesia (abnormal sensations). Pronounced low blood pressure and sinus bradycardia develop. In severe intoxication, loss of coordination and progressive muscular weakness result. Extrasystoles (a premature contraction of the heart that is independent of the normal rhythm and arises in response to an impulse in some part of the heart other than the sinoatrial node; called also premature beat) and ventricular tachycardia (an abnormally rapid ventricular rhythm with aberrant ventricular excitation, usually in excess of 150 per minute) with both atrioventricular and intraventricular conduction disturbances also may occur. Convulsions are reported occasionally.

Associated Foods

Grayanotoxin poisoning most commonly results from the ingestion of grayanotoxin-contaminated honey, although it may result from the ingestion of the leaves, flowers, and nectar of rhododendrons. Not all rhododendrons produce grayanotoxins. Rhododendron ponticum grows extensively on the mountains of the eastern Black Sea area of Turkey. This species has been associated with honey poisoning since 401 BC. A number of toxin species are native to the United States. Of particular importance are the western azalea (*Rhododendron occidentale*) found from Oregon to southern California, the California rosebay (*Rhododendron macrophyllum*) found from British Columbia to central California, and *Rhododendron albiflorum* found from British Columbia to Oregon and in Colorado. In the eastern half of the United States grayanotoxin-contaminated honey may be derived from other members of the botanical family Ericaceae, to which rhododendrons belong. Mountain laurel (*Kalmia latifolia*) and sheep laurel (*Kalmia angustifolia*) are probably the most important sources of the toxin.

Relative Frequency of Disease

Grayanotoxin poisoning in humans is rare. However, cases of honey intoxication should be anticipated everywhere. Some may be ascribed to a increase consumption of imported honey. Others may result from the ingestion of unprocessed honey with the increased desire of natural foods in the American diet.

Target Population

All people are believed to be susceptible to honey intoxication. The increased desire of the American public for natural (unprocessed) foods, may result in more cases of grayanotoxin poisoning. Individuals who obtain honey from farmers who may have only a few hives are at increased risk. The pooling of massive quantities of honey during commercial processing generally dilutes any toxic substance.

Analysis in Foods

The grayanotoxins can be isolated from the suspect commodity by typical extraction procedures for naturally occurring terpenes. The toxins are identified by thin layer chromatography.

Selected Outbreaks

Several cases of grayanotoxin poisonings in humans have been documented in the 1980s. These reports come from Turkey and Austria. The Austrian case resulted from the consumption of honey that was brought back from a visit to Turkey. From 1984 to 1986, 16 patients were treated for honey intoxication in Turkey. The symptoms started approximately 1 hour after 50 g of honey was consumed. In an average of 24 hours, all of the patients recovered. The case in Austria resulted in cardiac arrhythmia, which required a temporal pacemaker to prevent further decrease in heart rate. After a few hours, pacemaker simulation was no longer needed. The Austrian case shows that with increased travel throughout the world, the risk of grayanotoxin poisoning is possible outside the areas of Ericaceae-dominated vegetation, namely, Turkey, Japan, Brazil, United States, Nepal, and British Columbia. In 1983 several British veterinarians reported a incident of grayanotoxin poisoning in goats. One of the four animals died. Post-mortem examination showed grayanotoxin in the rumen contents.

For more information on recent outbreaks see the *Morbidity and Mortality Weekly Reports* from CDC.

Part Three

The Consumer's Role in Food Safety

Chapter 35

Home-Based Food-Borne Illness

When several members of a household come down with sudden, severe diarrhea and vomiting, intestinal flu is often considered the likely culprit. But food poisoning may be another consideration.

A true diagnosis is often never made because the ill people recover without having to see a doctor.

Health experts believe this is a common situation in households across the country, and because a doctor is often not seen for this kind of illness, the incidence of food-borne illness is not really known.

A task force of the Council for Agricultural Science and Technology, a private organization of food science groups, estimated in 1994 that 6.5 million to 33 million cases of food-borne illness occur in the United States each year. While many reported cases stem from food prepared by commercial or institutional establishments, sporadic cases and small outbreaks in homes are considered to be far more common, according to the April 1995 issue of Food Technology.

Cases of home-based food-borne illness may become a bigger problem, some food safety experts say, partly because today's busy family may not be as familiar with food safety issues as more home-focused families of past generations.

A 1993 FDA survey found that men respondents tended to be less safe about food practices than women respondents and that respondents younger than 40 tended to be less safe than those over 40.

For example, when asked if they believed that cooked food left at room temperature overnight is safe to eat without reheating—a very

1995 *FDA Consumer*, Food and Drug Administration.

unsafe practice—12 percent of the men respondents (but only 5 percent of the women respondents) said yes.

And, in looking at age differences, the survey found that nearly 40 percent of respondents younger than 40 indicated they did not adequately wash cutting boards, while only 25 percent of those 60 and over indicated the same.

The increased use of convenience foods, which often are preserved with special chemicals and processes, also complicates today's home food safety practices, said Robert Buchanan, Ph.D., lead scientist for FDA's food safety initiative. These foods, such as TV dinners, which are specially preserved, give consumers a false idea that equivalent home-cooked foods are equally safe, he said.

To curb the problem, food safety experts recommend food safety education that emphasizes the principles of HACCP (Hazard Analysis Critical Control Point), a new food safety procedure that many food companies are now incorporating into their manufacturing processes. Unlike past practices, HACCP focuses on preventing food-borne hazards, such as microbial contamination, by identifying points at which hazardous materials can be introduced into the food and then monitoring these potential problem areas. (See HACCP: Patrolling for Food Hazards in the January-February 1995 FDA Consumer.)

"It's mainly taking a common-sense approach towards food safety in the home," said Buchanan. "Basically, consumers need to make sure they're not defeating the system by contaminating the product."

More Information

FDA's Office of Consumer Affairs
HFE-88
Rockville, MD 20857

FDA Consumer Information Line
(1-800) 532-4440
(301) 827-4420 in the Washington, D.C. area
10 a.m. to 4 p.m. Eastern time, Monday through Friday

FDA Seafood Hotline
(1-800) FDA-4010
(202) 205-4314 in the Washington, D.C., area
24 hours a day

USDA's Meat and Poultry Hotline
(1-800) 535-4555
(202) 720-3333 in the Washington, D.C., area
Recorded messages available 24 hours a day. Home economists and registered dietitians available 10 a.m. to 4 p.m. Eastern time, Monday through Friday.

Also check with:

- your supermarket or its consumer affairs department
- your local county extension home economist
- local health departments
- food manufacturers

Food safety educators may contact:

Foodborne Illness Education Information Center
Food and Nutrition Information Center
National Agricultural Library/USDA
Beltsville, MD 20705-2351
Facsimile (301) 504-6409
E-mail: croberts@nalusda.gov

— by Paula Kurtzweil

Paula Kurtzweil is a member of FDA's public affairs staff.

Chapter 36

Can Your Kitchen Pass the Food Safety Test?

What comes to mind when you think of a clean kitchen? Shiny waxed floors? Gleaming stainless steel sinks? Spotless counters and neatly arranged cupboards?

They can help, but a truly "clean" kitchen—that is, one that ensures safe food—relies on more than just looks: It also depends on safe food practices.

In the home, food safety concerns revolve around three main functions: food storage, food handling, and cooking. To see how well you're doing in each, take this quiz, and then read on to learn how you can make the meals and snacks from your kitchen the safest possible.

Quiz

Choose the answer that best describes the practice in your household, whether or not you are the primary food handler.

1. The temperature of the refrigerator in my home is:
   a. 50 degrees Fahrenheit (10 degrees Celsius)
   b. 41 F (5° C)
   c. I don't know; I've never measured it.

2. The last time we had leftover cooked stew or other food with meat, chicken or fish, the food was:

1995 *FDA Consumer,* Food and Drug Administration.

a. cooled to room temperature, then put in the refrigerator

b. put in the refrigerator immediately after the food was served

c. left at room temperature overnight or longer

3. The last time the kitchen sink drain, disposal and connecting pipe in my home were sanitized was:

a. last night

b. several weeks ago

c. can't remember

4. If a cutting board is used in my home to cut raw meat, poultry or fish and it is going to be used to chop another food, the board is:

a. reused as is

b. wiped with a damp cloth

c. washed with soap and hot water

d. washed with soap and hot water and then sanitized

5. The last time we had hamburgers in my home, I ate mine:

a. rare

b. medium

c. well-done

6. The last time there was cookie dough in my home, the dough was:

a. made with raw eggs, and I sampled some of it

b. store-bought, and I sampled some of it

c. not sampled until baked

7. I clean my kitchen counters and other surfaces that come in contact with food with:

a. water

b. hot water and soap

c. hot water and soap, then bleach solution

d. hot water and soap, then commercial sanitizing agent

8. When dishes are washed in my home, they are:

a. cleaned by an automatic dishwasher and then air-dried

b. left to soak in the sink for several hours and then washed with soap in the same water

    c. washed right away with hot water and soap in the sink
       and then air-dried

    d. washed right away with hot water and soap in the sink
       and immediately towel-dried

9.   The last time I handled raw meat, poultry or fish, I cleaned
my hands afterwards by:
    a. wiping them on a towel
    b. rinsing them under hot, cold or warm tap water
    c. washing with soap and warm water

10.   Meat, poultry and fish products are defrosted in my home by:
    a. setting them on the counter
    b. placing them in the refrigerator
    c. microwaving

11.   When I buy fresh seafood, I:
    a. buy only fish that's refrigerated or well iced
    b. take it home immediately and put it in the refrigerator
    c. sometimes buy it straight out of a local fisher's creel

12.   I realize people, including myself, should be especially careful
about not eating raw seafood, if they have:
    a. diabetes
    b. HIV infection
    c. cancer
    d. liver disease

Answers

    1.   Refrigerators should stay at 41 F (5° C) or less, so if you chose answer B, give yourself two points. If you didn't, you're not alone. According to Robert Buchanan, Ph.D., food safety initiative lead scientist in the Food and Drug Administration's Center for Food Safety and Applied Nutrition, many people overlook the importance of maintaining an appropriate refrigerator temperature.

    "According to surveys, in many households, the refrigerator temperature is above 50 degrees (10° C)," he said. His advice: Measure the temperature with a thermometer and, if needed, adjust the refrigerator's temperature control dial.

    A temperature of 41 F (5° C) or less is important because it slows the growth of most bacteria. The temperature won't kill the bacteria, but it will keep them from multiplying, and the fewer there are, the less likely you are to get sick from them. Freezing at zero F (minus 18° C) or less stops bacterial growth (although it won't kill all bacteria already present).

2. Answer B is the best practice; give yourself two points if you picked it.

Hot foods should be refrigerated as soon as possible within two hours after cooking. But don't keep the food if it's been standing out for more than two hours. Don't taste test it, either. Even a small amount of contaminated food can cause illness.

Date leftovers so they can be used within a safe time. Generally, they remain safe when refrigerated for three to five days. If in doubt, throw it out, said FDA microbiologist Kelly Bunning, Ph.D., also with FDA's food safety initiative. "It's not worth a food-borne illness for the small amount of food usually involved."

3. If answer A best describes your household's practice, give yourself two points. Give yourself one point if you chose B.

According to FDA's John Guzewich epidemiologist on FDA's food safety initiative team, the kitchen sink drain, disposal and connecting pipe are often overlooked, but they should be sanitized periodically by pouring down the sink a solution of 1 teaspoon (5 milliliters) of chlorine bleach in 1 quart (about 1 liter) of water or a solution of commercial kitchen cleaning agent made according to product directions. Food particles get trapped in the drain and disposal and, along with the moistness, create an ideal environment for bacterial growth.

4. If answer D best describes your household's practice, give yourself two points.

If you picked A, you're violating an important food safety rule: Never allow raw meat, poultry and fish to come in contact with other foods. Answer B isn't good, either. Improper washing, such as with a damp cloth, will not remove bacteria. And washing only with soap and water may not do the job, either.

5. Give yourself two points if you picked answer C.

If you don't have a meat thermometer, there are other ways to determine whether seafood is done:

- For fish, slip the point of a sharp knife into the flesh and pull aside. The edges should be opaque and the center slightly translucent with flakes beginning to separate. Let the fish stand three to four minutes to finish cooking.

- For shrimp, lobster and scallops, check color. Shrimp and lobster and scallops, red and the flesh becomes pearly opaque. Scallops turn milky white or opaque and firm.

- For clams, mussels and oysters, watch for the point at which their shells open. Boil three to five minutes longer. Throw out those that stay closed. When using the microwave, rotate the dish several times to ensure even cooking. Follow recommended standing times. After the standing time is completed, check the seafood in several spots with a meat thermometer to be sure the product has reached the proper temperature.

6. If you answered A, you may be putting yourself at risk for infection with *Salmonella enteritidis,* a bacterium that can be in shell eggs. Cooking the egg or egg-containing food product to an internal temperature of at least 145° F (63° C) kills the bacteria. So answer C—eating the baked product—will earn you two points.

You'll get two points for answer B, also. Foods containing raw eggs, such as homemade ice cream, cake batter, mayonnaise, and eggnog, carry a Salmonella risk, but their commercial counterparts don't. Commercial products are made with pasteurized eggs; that is, eggs that have been heated sufficiently to kill bacteria, and also may contain an acidifying agent that kills the bacteria. Commercial preparations of cookie dough are not a food hazard.

If you want to sample homemade dough or batter or eat other foods with raw-egg-containing products, consider substituting pasteurized eggs for raw eggs. Pasteurized eggs are usually sold in the grocer's refrigerated dairy case.

Some other tips to ensure egg safety:

- Buy only refrigerated eggs, and keep them refrigerated until you are ready to cook and serve them.

- Cook eggs thoroughly until both the yolk and white are firm, not runny, and scramble until there is no visible liquid egg.

- Cook pasta dishes and stuffings that contain eggs thoroughly.

7. Answers C or D will earn you two points each; answer B, one point. According to FDA's Guzewich, bleach and commercial kitchen cleaning agents are the best sanitizers—provided they're diluted according to product directions. They're the most effective at getting rid of bacteria. Hot water and soap does a good job too, but may not kill all strains of bacteria. Water may get rid of visible dirt but not bacteria.

Also, be sure to keep dishcloths and sponges clean because, when wet, these materials harbor bacteria and may promote their growth.

8. Answers A and C are worth two points each. There are potential problems with B and D. When you let dishes sit in water for a long time, it "creates a soup," FDA's Buchanan said. "The food left on the dish contributes nutrients for bacteria, so the bacteria will multiply." When washing dishes by hand, he said, it's best to wash them all within two hours. Also, it's best to air-dry them so you don't handle them while they're wet.

9. The only correct practice is answer C. Give yourself two points if you picked it.

Wash hands with warm water and soap for at least 20 seconds before and after handling food, especially raw meat, poultry and fish. If you have an infection or cut on your hands, wear rubber or plastic gloves. Wash gloved hands just as often as bare hands because the gloves can pick up bacteria. (However, when washing gloved hands, you don't need to take off your gloves and wash your bare hands, too.)

10. Give yourself two points if you picked B or C. Food safety experts recommend thawing foods in the refrigerator or the microwave oven or putting the package in a water-tight plastic bag submerged in cold water and changing the water every 30 minutes. Gradual defrosting overnight is best because it helps maintain quality.

When microwaving, follow package directions. Leave about 2 inches (about 5 centimeters) between the food and the inside surface of the microwave to allow heat to circulate. Smaller items will defrost more evenly than larger pieces of food. Foods defrosted in the microwave oven should be cooked immediately after thawing.

Do not thaw meat, poultry and fish products on the counter or in the sink without cold water; bacteria can multiply rapidly at room temperature. Marinate food in the refrigerator, not on the counter. Discard the marinade after use because it contains raw juices, which may harbor bacteria. If you want to use the marinade as a dip or sauce, reserve a portion before adding raw food.

11. A and B are correct. Give yourself two points for either.

When buying fresh seafood, buy only from reputable dealers who keep their products refrigerated or properly iced. Be wary, for example, of vendors selling fish out of their creel (canvas bag) or out of the back of their truck.

Once you buy the seafood, immediately put it on ice, in the refrigerator or in the freezer. Some other tips for choosing safe seafood:

- Don't buy cooked seafood, such as shrimp, crabs or smoked fish, if displayed in the same case as raw fish. Cross-contamination can occur. Or, at least, make sure the raw fish is on a level lower than the cooked fish so that the raw fish juices don't flow onto the cooked items and contaminate them.

- Don't buy frozen seafood if the packages are open, torn or crushed on the edges. Avoid packages that are above the frost line in the store's freezer. If the package cover is transparent, look for signs of frost or ice crystals. This could mean that the fish has either been stored for a long time or thawed and refrozen.

- Recreational fishers who plan to eat their catch should follow state and local government advisories about fishing areas and eating fish from certain areas.

- As with meat and poultry, if seafood will be used within two days after purchase, store it in the coldest part of the refrigerator, usually under the freezer compartment or in a special "meat keeper." Avoid packing it in tightly with other items; allow air to circulate freely around the package. Otherwise, wrap the food tightly in moisture-proof freezer paper or foil to protect it from air leaks and store in the freezer.

- Discard shellfish, such as lobsters, crabs, oysters, clams and mussels, if they die during storage or if their shells crack or break. Live shellfish close up when the shell is tapped.

12. If you are under treatment for any of these diseases, as well as several others, you should avoid raw seafood. Give yourself two points for knowing one or more of the risky conditions.

People with certain diseases and conditions need to be especially careful because their diseases or the medicine they take may put them at risk for serious illness or death from contaminated seafood.

These conditions include:

- liver disease, either from excessive alcohol use, viral hepatitis, or other causes

- hemochromatosis, an iron disorder

- diabetes

- stomach problems, including previous stomach surgery and low stomach acid (for example, from antacid use)

- cancer

- immune disorders, including HIV infection

- long-term steroid use, as for asthma and arthritis

Older adults also may be at increased risk because they more often have these conditions.

People with these diseases or conditions should never eat raw seafood—only seafood that has been thoroughly cooked.

Rating Your Home's Food Practices

24 points: Feel confident about the safety of foods served in your home.

12 to 23 points: Reexamine food safety practices in your home. Some key rules are being violated.

11 points or below: Take steps immediately to correct food handling, storage and cooking techniques used in your home. Current practices are putting you and other members of your household in danger of food-borne illness.

— by Paula Kurtzweil

Paula Kurtzweil is a member of FDA's public affairs staff.

Chapter 37

Sponges, Sinks, and Rags

Think household germs, and chances are you'll think of the bathroom. Yet when scientists from the University of Arizona in Tucson sample surfaces from kitchens and bathrooms in the same house, "consistently, kitchens come up dirtier," notes microbiologist Carlos Enriquez. This trend holds even for disease-causing germs spread by fecal contamination, such as the *Escherichia coli* coliform bacteria. "We have swabbed the toilet rim, for instance, and seldom do we find fecal coliform bacteria there, surprising as that may sound," he observes. Enter the kitchen, though, and they're everywhere—in the sponges, dish towels, sink, even on countertops. "So my boss usually jokes about it being safer eating dinner in the bathroom," he says.

But kitchen pathogens are no laughing matter. In the United States, the diseases they cause kill an estimated 9,000 persons each year-mostly the very young, the very old, and those with severely weakened immune systems. The cost of treating foodborne infections ranges from $5 billion to $22 billion annually, according to an analysis released in May by the U.S. General Accounting Office.

Though state and federal agencies compile records on widespread or highly publicized cases—like the *E. coli* deaths traced to hamburger served at Jack-in-the-Box restaurants in early 1993—they have little information on cases involving just one or two individuals, especially when the ensuing stomach cramps, vomiting, or diarrhea don't lead to hospitalization. However, when researchers have attempted to tally homespun outbreaks, the numbers have proved staggering, notes food safety expert Elizabeth Scott of Newton, Mass.

In the January *Journal of Applied Bacteriology*, she reviewed European data on disease that could be traced to food eaten at home. For 1989 to 1991 in England and Wales, for instance, 86 percent of the 2,766 reported outbreaks of *salmonella* infection involving one or more persons appeared to stem from household exposure.

Says Enriquez, these data indicate that "even though we usually feel more secure eating at home, it doesn't necessarily mean it's safer." He and researchers in a few other labs around the country are now investigating where kitchen bugs lurk, with an eye toward making home cooking safer.

Sponges provide an ideal way to spread disease, a discovery the Arizona researchers stumbled upon while swabbing kitchen surfaces daily in several homes.

Bacteria tend to be concentrated in the sink, its drain, and the sponge, Enriquez and his colleagues found. In one home they examined, however, everything from the countertops to refrigerator handles bore consistently heavy contamination-until the sixth day, when most surfaces suddenly turned up virtually germfree. It turned out the family had simply begun using a new sponge.

That was a few years ago. At the American Society for Microbiology meeting in New Orleans last May, Enriquez and his coworkers reported finding that most of the 75 dishrags and 325 sponges from home kitchens that they have sampled harbor large numbers of virulent bacteria (SN: 5/25/96, p. 326), including *E. coli* and strains of *Salmonella, Pseudomonas*, and *Staphylococcus*.

They measure bacteria in colony-forming units, one or more cells that, when cultured, generates a clump of bacteria. In wet areas around the sink, and especially its drain, Enriquez's group has measured up to 10,000 colony-forming units per milliliter of moisture sampled. "And we've found up to 10 million colony-forming units in 1 ml of the liquid wrung from a sponge," he told Science News.

"Initially, we were surprised," he says. In retrospect, the microbiologists realized that continually moist cellulose sponges provide "a very hospitable environment" for bacteria. Key to their survival is a surface easy to cling to, a steady supply of nutrients—even microscopic scraps of food—and moisture.

If a sponge stays moist, the number of live microbes doesn't decrease for 2 weeks. Bacteria can even survive for at least 2 days, Enriquez finds, in a damp sponge gradually drying in the air.

On dry surfaces, resident bacteria survive no more than a few hours. However, Enriquez points out, that's long enough to infect another source of food, or a person's hands during meal preparation.

Though bacteria may love sponges, they happily colonize even stainless steel, notes Edmund A. Zottola of the University of Minnesota in St. Paul. Metal that appears smooth to the naked eye is, from a microbe's perspective, "full of all kinds of nooks and crannies, canyons, gullies, and hills," he observes.

Whenever bacteria find a site harboring moisture and food, he says, "they will set up housekeeping and grow."

His studies have shown that if they aren't sent packing quickly, the microbes produce an organic goo with threadlike tendrils "that literally cements the cells to the surface." This allows them to weather the elements, fast-flowing sprays of water, a little rubbing, or a weak detergent solution. Eventually, unrelated families of microbes move in. The resulting cosmopolitan community forms biofilms that further protect its inhabitants.

Cutting boards, with their accumulations of scars, also prove hospitable to bacteria. About 4 years ago, Philip H. Kass and his colleagues at the University of California, Davis found that victims of sporadic salmonellosis—infections not linked to large outbreaks—were more likely to use plastic cutting boards than wooden ones. At about the same time, microbiologist Dean O. Cliver, then at the University of Wisconsin in Madison, began investigating cutting board hygiene (SN: 2/6/93, p. 84). In the January 1994 *Journal of Food Protection*, Cliver and his colleagues reported that it is easier to recover live bacteria from a plastic board than a wooden one. In the wood, germs hide out in the millimeter or so below the surface.

More recently, Carl A. Batt of Cornell University and his colleagues discovered that the differences between wooden and plastic boards depend on how moist they are. "If the wood board is somewhat wet and then you apply bacteria to it, you can pull those bacteria off as easily as you can from plastic," he observes. "But a dry wood board absorbs moisture and draws the bacteria into its pores by capillary action." These findings are slated for publication in Food Microbiology.

Cliver's group is now investigating whether cutting into the surface of either type of cutting board can retrieve and transport previously hidden bugs to other foods. So far, Cliver told Science News, knives are "getting more bacteria out of knife-scarred plastic boards than out of knife- scarred wood boards."

The good news is that kitchen germs can usually be removed by some method of cleansing. On metal surfaces, Zottola says, detergent dissolves the food and microbial material. A good rubbing then forcibly evicts most of the squatters.

A follow-up, sanitizing rinse—such as a solution of dilute bleach (hypochlorous acid)—will annihilate even the most tenacious hangers-on, he's found. To deter recolonization, the cleansed surfaces must stay dry. Wood requires a different sterilization regime, Zottola points out, because its organic building blocks will react with bleach, rendering the disinfectant unavailable for killing germs. As a result, cooks have had to be satisfied with just bathing their wooden cutting boards.

In the January 1994 *Journal of Food Protection*, Cliver and his colleagues showed that it is possible, using soap and water, to hand scrub microbes from the surface of new or used wooden cutting boards and from new plastic ones.

Plastic boards that bore the knife scars of use, however, proved resistant to decontamination by hand washing.

Bacteria below the surface of a wooden board are untouched by hand scrubbing and can remain alive at least several hours. Even though at that location they can't contaminate other foods that may contact the board, it remains prudent to kill them, says Cliver, now at UC-Davis.

In a pair of papers to be published in the *Journal of Food Protection*, Cliver and Paul K. Park report success in annihilating *E. coli* and *Staphylococcus aureus* with microwave heating. They contaminated wooden cutting boards with 1 billion colony-forming units per 25 square centimeters of surface and then cooked the boards on high heat in an 800- watt home microwave oven.

After 10 minutes, a medium-sized board emerged bone dry-and free of live microbes both on and below the surface. Wetting the board speeded the killing, suggesting that the microbes probably boiled to death.

The microwave can also disinfect other kitchen items. Sterilizing dry cellulose sponges took a mere 30 seconds, while wet sponges took 1 minute. Cotton dishrags required 30 seconds when dry but 3 minutes when wet. No amount of microwaving disinfected plastic boards. That's not surprising, Cliver notes, since their surfaces never achieved cell-killing temperatures. However, studies by others have shown that the normal cycle in a dishwasher can sterilize even well-used plastic boards.

Whether you use wood or plastic cutting boards becomes unimportant at home if you are into cleaning and sanitizing-as all cooks should

212

be, Batt argues. Many people, however, aren't. A study published last year by scientists at the Food and Drug Administration found that 26 percent of U.S. consumers don't bother to clean cutting boards after using them for raw meat or chicken. Moreover, many food safety specialists, such as microbiologist Charles E. Benson of the University of Pennsylvania School of Veterinary Medicine in Kennett Square, note that few publications specifically focus on the home kitchen. The few that do, Benson says, generally offer suggestions "based on no concrete evidence."

With a growing incidence of foodborne disease in the United States and limited consumer knowledge, Theodore P. Labuza suspects that the next wave of kitchen safety technologies will be self-disinfecting appliances, packaging, and building materials. A food safety engineer at the University of Minnesota, he sees particular promise in what he has termed "active" surfaces.

Today, he notes, one can buy sponges with bacteria-killing compounds built into the cellulose. There's no reason similar agents couldn't be engineered into countertops, he notes, or the paints used on the inside of refrigerators. Antimicrobial cutting boards are already being sold, and the Japanese are marketing plastic bags that claim to emit germ-killing radiation. When it comes to food safety, "research paradigm shifts need to occur for the 21st century," he says. Making home kitchens self-disinfecting, he argues, "is certainly one of them."

Chapter 38

Slow Cooker Safety

Opening the front door on a cold winter evening and being greeted by the inviting smells of beef stew or chicken noodle soup wafting from a slow cooker can be a diner's dream come true. But winter is not the only time a slow cooker is useful. In the summer, using this small appliance can avoid introducing heat from a hot oven. At any time of year, a slow cooker can make life a little more convenient because by planning ahead, you save time later. And it takes less electricity to use a slow cooker rather than an oven.

Is a Slow Cooker Safe?

Yes, the slow cooker, a countertop appliance, cooks foods slowly at a low temperature—generally between 170° and 280° F. The low heat helps less expensive, leaner cuts of meat become tender and shrink less.

The direct heat from the pot, lengthy cooking and steam created within the tightly covered container combine to destroy bacteria and make the slow cooker a safe process for cooking foods.

Safe Beginnings

Begin with a clean cooker, clean utensils and a clean work area. Wash hands before and during food preparation.

Consumer Education and Information, December 1994; Food Safety and Inspection Service; United States Department of Agriculture, Washington, D.C. 20250-3700.

Keep perishable foods refrigerated until preparation time. If you cut up meat and vegetables in advance, store them separately in the refrigerator. The slow cooker may take several hours to reach a safe, bacteria-killing temperature. Constant refrigeration assures that bacteria, which multiply rapidly at room temperature, won't get a "head start" during the first few hours of cooking.

Thaw and Cut Up Ingredients

Always defrost meat or poultry before putting it into a slow cooker. Choose to make foods with a high moisture content such as chili, soup, stew or spaghetti sauce.

Cut food into chunks or small pieces to ensure thorough cooking. Do not use the slow cooker for large pieces like a roast or whole chicken because the food will cook so slowly it could remain in the bacterial "danger zone" too long.

Use the Right Amount of Food

Fill cooker no less than half full and no more than two-thirds full. Vegetables cook slower than meat and poultry in a slow cooker so if using them, put vegetables in first, at the bottom and around sides of the utensil. Then add meat and cover the food with liquid such as broth, water or barbecue sauce. Keep the lid in place, removing only to stir the food or check for doneness.

Settings

Most cookers have two or more settings. Foods take different times to cook depending upon the setting used. Certainly, foods will cook faster on high than on low. However, for all-day cooking or for less-tender cuts, you may want to use the low setting.

If possible, turn the cooker on the highest setting for the first hour of cooking time and then to low or the setting called for in your recipe. However, it's safe to cook foods on low the entire time—if you're leaving for work, for example, and preparation time is limited.

While food is cooking and once it's done, food will stay safe as long as the cooker is operating.

Power Out

If you are not at home during the entire slow-cooking process and the power goes out, throw away the food even if it looks done.

If you are at home, finish cooking the ingredients immediately by some other means: on a gas stove, on the outdoor grill or at a house where the power is on. When you are at home, and if the food was completely cooked before the power went out, the food should remain safe up to two hours in the cooker with the power off.

Handling Leftovers

Store leftovers in shallow covered containers and refrigerate within two hours after cooking is finished. Reheating leftovers in a slow cooker is not recommended. However, cooked food can be brought to steaming on the stove top or in a microwave oven and then put into a preheated slow cooker to keep hot for serving.

For additional food safety information about meat, poultry or eggs, call the toll-free USDA Meat and Poultry Hotline at 1 (800) 535-4555. It is staffed by home economists from 10 a.m. to 4 p.m. ET year round. An extensive selection of food safety recordings can be heard 24 hours a day using a touch-tone phone. The media may call Bessie Berry, Acting Director, USDA Meat and Poultry Hotline, at (202) 720-5604.

For Further Information Contact:

FSIS Food Safety Education and Communications Staff
Meat and Poultry Hotline:
1-800-535-4555 (Tollfree Nationwide)
(202) 720-3333 (Washington, DC area)
1-800-256-7072 (TDD/TTY)

Chapter 39

Freezing

Foods in the freezer—are they safe? Every year, thousands of callers to the USDA Meat and Poultry Hotline aren't sure about the safety of items stored in their own home freezers. The confusion seems to be based on the fact that few people understand how freezing protects food. Here is some information on how to freeze food safely and how long to keep it.

What Can You Freeze?

You can freeze almost any foods. Some exceptions are cans of foods or eggs in shells. However, once the food (such as a ham) is out of the can, you may freeze it.

Being able to freeze food and being pleased with the quality after defrosting are two different things. Some foods simply don't freeze well at all. Examples are mayonnaise, cream sauce and lettuce. Raw meat and poultry maintain their quality longer than their cooked counterparts because moisture is lost during cooking.

Is Frozen Food Safe?

Food stored constantly at 0° F will always be safe. Only the quality suffers with lengthy freezer storage. Freezing keeps food safe by slowing the movement of molecules, causing microbes to enter a dormant

Food Safety and Inspection Service; United States Department of Agriculture, Washington, D.C. 20250-3700.

stage. Freezing preserves food for extended periods because it prevents the growth of microorganisms that cause both food spoilage and foodborne illness.

Does Freezing Destroy Bacteria and Parasites?

Freezing to 0° F inactivates any microbes—bacteria, yeasts and molds—present in food. Once thawed, however, these microbes can again become active, multiplying under the right conditions to levels that can lead to foodborne illness. Since they will then grow at about the same rate as microorganisms on fresh food, you must handle thawed items as you would any perishable. Thorough cooking will destroy bacteria.

Trichina and other parasites can be destroyed by sub-zero freezing temperatures. However, very strict government-supervised conditions must be met. It is not recommended to rely on home freezing to destroy trichina. Thorough cooking will destroy all parasites.

Freshness and Quality

Freshness and quality at the time of freezing affect the condition of frozen foods. If frozen at peak quality, foods emerge tasting better than foods frozen near the end of their useful life. So freeze items you won't use quickly sooner rather than later. Store all foods at 0° F or lower to retain vitamin content, color, flavor and texture.

Nutrient Retention

The freezing process itself does not destroy nutrients. In meat and poultry products, there is little change in nutrient value during freezer storage.

Enzymes

Enzyme activity can lead to the deterioration of foods quality. Enzymes present in animals, vegetables and fruit promote chemical reactions, such as ripening. Freezing only slows the enzyme activity that takes place in foods. It does not halt these reactions which continue after harvesting. Enzyme activity does not harm frozen meats or fish and is neutralized by the acids in frozen fruits. But most vegetables that freeze well are low acid and require a brief, partial cooking to prevent deterioration. This is called "blanching." For successful freezing, blanch or partially cook vegetables in boiling water or in a microwave oven. Then rapidly chill the vegetables prior to freezing and storage. Consult a cookbook for timing.

Packaging

Proper packaging helps maintain quality and prevent "freezer burn." It is safe to freeze meat or poultry directly in its supermarket wrapping but this type of wrap is permeable to air. Unless you will be using the food in a month or two, overwrap these packages as you would any food for long-term storage using airtight heavy-duty foil, plastic wrap or freezer paper, or place the package inside a plastic bag. Use these materials or airtight freezer containers to repackage family packs into smaller amounts or freeze foods from opened packages. It is not necessary to rinse meat and poultry before freezing. Freeze unopened vacuum packages as is. If you notice that a package has accidentally torn or has opened while food is in the freezer, it is still safe to use; merely overwrap or rewrap it.

Freezer Burn

Freezer burn does not make food unsafe, merely dry in spots. It appears as grayish-brown leathery spots and is caused by air reaching the surface of the food. Cut freezer-burned portions away either before or after cooking the food. Heavily freezer-burned foods may have to be discarded for quality reasons.

Color Changes

Color changes can occur in frozen foods. The bright red color of meat as purchased usually turns dark or pale brown depending on its variety. This may be due to lack of oxygen, freezer burn or abnormally long storage.

Freezing doesn't usually cause color changes in poultry. However, the bones and the meat near them can become dark. Bone darkening results when pigment seeps through the porous bones of young poultry into the surrounding tissues when the poultry meat is frozen and thawed.

The dulling of color in frozen vegetables and cooked foods is usually the result of excessive drying due to improper packaging or overlengthy storage.

Freeze Rapidly

Freeze food as fast as possible to maintain its quality. Rapid freezing prevents undesirable large ice crystals from forming throughout the product because the molecules don't have time to take their positions in the characteristic six-sided snowflake. Slow freezing creates large, disruptive ice crystals. During thawing, they damage the cells and dissolve emulsions. This causes meat to "drip"—lose juiciness. Emulsions such as mayonnaise or cream will separate and appear curdled.

Ideally, a food 2-inches thick should freeze completely in about 2 hours. If your home freezer has a "quick-freeze" shelf, use it. Never stack packages to be frozen. Instead, spread them out in one layer on various shelves, stacking them only after frozen solid.

Refrigerator-Freezers

If a refrigerator freezing compartment can't maintain zero degrees or if the door is opened frequently, use it for short-term food storage. Eat those foods as soon as possible for best quality. Use a free-standing freezer set at 0° F or below for long-term storage of frozen foods. And keep a thermometer in your freezing compartment or freezer to check the temperature.

Length of Time

Because freezing keeps food safe almost indefinitely, recommended storage times are for quality only. Refer to the freezer storage chart at the end of this chapter or see "A Quick Consumer Guide to Safe Food Handling" which lists optimum freezing times for best quality.

If a food is not listed on the chart, you may determine its quality after defrosting. First check the odor. Some foods will develop a rancid or off odor when frozen too long and should be discarded. Some may not look picture perfect or be of high enough quality to serve alone but may be edible; use them to make soups or stews. Cook raw food and if you like the taste and texture, use it.

Safe Defrosting

Never defrost foods in a garage, basement, car, dishwasher or plastic garbage bag; out on the kitchen counter, outdoors or on the porch. These methods can leave your foods unsafe to eat.

There are three safe ways to defrost food: in the refrigerator, in cold water or in the microwave. It's best to plan ahead for slow, safe thawing in the refrigerator. Small items may defrost overnight; most foods require a day or two. And large items like turkeys may take longer—one day for each 5 pounds of weight.

For faster defrosting, place food in a leakproof plastic bag and immerse it in cold water. (If the bag leaks, bacteria from the air or surrounding environment could be introduced into the food. Tissues can also absorb water like a sponge, resulting in a watery product.) Check the water frequently to be sure it stays cold. Change the water every 30 minutes. After thawing, refrigerate the food until ready to use.

When microwave-defrosting food, plan to cook it immediately after thawing because some areas of the food may become warm and begin to cook during microwaving. Holding partially cooked food is not recommended because any bacteria present wouldn't have been destroyed.

Refreezing

Once food is thawed in the refrigerator, it is safe to refreeze it without cooking, although there may be a loss of quality due to the moisture lost through defrosting. After cooking raw foods which were previously frozen, it is safe to freeze the cooked foods. And if previously cooked foods are thawed in the refrigerator, you may refreeze the unused portion.

If you purchase previously frozen meat, poultry or fish at a retail store, you can refreeze if it has been handled properly.

Cooking Frozen Foods

Raw or cooked meat, poultry or casseroles can be cooked or re-heated from the frozen state. However, it will take approximately one and a half times the usual cooking time for food which has been thawed. Remember to discard any wrapping or absorbent paper from meat or poultry.

When cooking whole poultry, remove the giblet pack from the cavity as soon as you can loosen it. Cook the giblets separately. Read the label on USDA-inspected frozen meat and poultry products. Some, such as pre-stuffed whole birds, MUST be cooked from the frozen state to ensure a safely cooked product.

Power Outage in Freezer

If there is a power outage, the freezer fails or if the freezer door has been left ajar by mistake, the food may still be safe to use. As long as a freezer with its door ajar is continuing to cool, the foods should stay safe overnight. If a repairman is on the way or it appears the power will be on soon, just don't open the freezer door.

A freezer full of food will usually keep about 2 days if the door is kept shut; a half-full freezer will last about a day. The freezing compartment in a refrigerator may not keep foods frozen as long. If the freezer is not full, quickly group packages together so they will retain the cold more effectively. Separate meat and poultry items from other foods so if they begin to thaw, their juices won't drip onto other foods.

For short term power outages—less than 6 hours—leave the door closed until the power returns. If the power is off for more than 6

Table 39.1. Freezer Storage Chart (0° F)

NOTE: Freezer storage is for quality only. Frozen foods remain safe indefinitely.

Item	Months
Bacon and Sausage	1 to 2
Casseroles	1 to 2
Egg whites or egg substitutes	12
Gravy, meat or poultry	2 to 3
Ham, Hotdogs and Lunchmeats	1 to 2
Meat, uncooked roasts	9
Meat, uncooked steaks or chops	4 to 6
Meat, uncooked ground	3 to 4
Meat, cooked	2 to 3
Poultry, uncooked whole	12
Poultry, uncooked parts	9
Poultry, uncooked giblets	3 to 4
Poultry, cooked	3 to 4
Soups and Stews	2 to 3
Wild game, uncooked	8 to 12

hours, you may want to put dry ice, block ice or bags of ice in the freezer, or transfer foods to a friend's freezer until power is restored. Use an appliance thermometer to monitor the temperature.

If it's freezing outside or if there's snow on the ground, that might seem like a good place to keep food frozen until the power comes on. However, foods stored in the great outdoors are exposed to the sun, environmental contamination, roaming animals and birds. So keep food indoors.

To determine the safety of foods when the power goes on, check their condition and temperature. If food is partly frozen, still has ice crystals or is as cold as if it were in a refrigerator (40° F), it is safe to refreeze or use. It's not necessary to cook raw foods before refreezing. Discard foods that have been warmer than 40° F for more than 2 hours. Discard any foods that have been contaminated by raw meat juices. Dispose of soft or melted ice cream for quality's sake.

Frozen Cans

Accidentally frozen cans, such as those left in a car or basement in sub-zero temperatures, can present health problems. If the cans are merely swollen—and you are sure the swelling was caused by freezing—the cans may still be usable. Let the can thaw in the refrigerator before opening. If the product doesn't look and/or smell normal, throw it out. DO NOT TASTE IT! However, if the product does look and/or smell normal, thoroughly cook the contents by boiling for 10 to 20 minutes right away. But if the seams have rusted or burst, throw the cans out immediately.

Frozen Eggs

Shell eggs should not be frozen. If an egg accidentally freezes and the shell cracked during freezing, discard the egg. Keep an uncracked egg frozen until needed; then thaw in the refrigerator. It can be hard cooked successfully but other uses may be limited. That's because freezing causes the yolk to become thick and syrupy so it will not flow like an unfrozen yolk or blend very well with the egg white or other ingredients.

More Information

For additional food safety information about meat, poultry or eggs, call the toll-free USDA Meat and Poultry Hotline at 1 (800) 535-4555.

It is staffed by home economists from 10 a.m. to 4 p.m. ET year round. An extensive selection of food safety recordings can be heard 24 hours a day using a touch-tone phone.

For Further Information Contact

FSIS Food Safety Education and Communications Staff
Meat and Poultry Hotline:
1-800-535-4555 (Tollfree Nationwide)

Chapter 40

Safe Food to Go

For bag lunches, picnics, or celebrations away from home, food can be kept safe if it is first handled and cooked safely. Then, keeping food cold while transporting and serving, as well as practicing safe grilling techniques, can prevent foodborne illness.

Beginning with Safe Food

Perishable food must be kept cold or frozen at the store and at home. In between, the food should be at room temperature or in the car as little time as possible. Then it must be kept cold or cooked and chilled. Food should not be out of the refrigerator or oven longer than 2 hours.

If cooking foods beforehand—such as turkey, ham, chicken, and vegetable or pasta salads—prepare them in plenty of time to thoroughly chill in the refrigerator. Divide large amounts of food into small containers for fast chilling and easier use. Keep cooked foods refrigerated until time to leave home.

Packing for Outings

If taking food away from home—on a picnic, for example—try to plan just the right amount of perishable foods to take. That way, you won't have to worry about the storage or safety of leftovers.

1998, Food Safety and Inspection Service; United States Department of Agriculture, Washington, D.C. 20250-3700.

Items which don't require refrigeration include fruits, vegetables, hard cheese, canned meat or fish, chips, bread, crackers, peanut butter, jelly, mustard, and pickles. You don't need to pack them in a cooler.

It's perfectly safe to store uncooked patties as well as raw steaks, ribs, chops, and raw poultry in the refrigerator for a day or so until ready to pack the cooler.

If marinating meat and poultry, store it in the refrigerator—not on the counter. If you plan to use some of the marinade as a sauce, reserve a portion before putting raw meat in it. Don't reuse the marinade from meat unless it's boiled first to destroy any bacteria that may have been on the raw meat.

Purchasing Take-Out Foods

If you're planning on purchasing take-out foods such as fried chicken or barbecued beef, eat them within 2 hours of pickup. Otherwise, buy cooked foods ahead of time to chill before packing them into the cooler.

Keeping Cold Food Cold

After estimating the amount of food which needs to be kept cold, pack an insulated cooler with sufficient ice or gel packs to keep the food at 40° F. Pack food right from the refrigerator or freezer into it.

Why? Bacteria grow and multiply rapidly in the danger zone between 40° F and 140° F (out of the refrigerator or before food begins to cook). So, food transported without an ice source or left out in the sun at a picnic won't stay safe long.

If packing a bag lunch or lunch box, it's fine to prepare the food the night before and store the packed lunch in the refrigerator.

To keep the lunch cool away from home, pack a small frozen gel pack or frozen juice box. Of course, if there's a refrigerator at work, store perishable items there upon arrival. Leftover perishables which have been kept refrigerated should be safe to take home. But once gel packs and other cold sources melt, perishables are not safe—discard them.

When taking food to a picnic, don't put the cooler in the trunk; carry it inside the air-conditioned car. At the picnic, keep the cooler in the shade. Keep the lid closed and avoid repeated openings. Replenish the ice if it melts.

Serving Food

Except when served, the food should be stored in a cooler. Just like a refrigerator at home when the power is off, the more times you open a cooler, the more cold air will escape. Once the ice melts, the cooler won't be able to keep food safe. Keep cold drinks in a separate cooler to avoid constantly opening the one containing perishable foods.

If you've packed cooked foods in several small containers, you can serve one and keep the others cold for second helpings. Leave raw meat in the cooler, too. When cooking it, remove from the cooler only the amount that will fit on the grill.

Grilling Safety

For safety and quality, the coals should be very hot before cooking food. For optimal heat, burn them 20 to 30 minutes or until they are lightly coated with ash. The USDA recommends against eating raw or undercooked ground beef since harmful bacteria could be present. To be sure bacteria are destroyed, cook hamburgers to 160° F on a meat thermometer. Large cuts of beef such as roasts may be cooked to 145° F for medium rare or to 160° F for medium. Cook ground poultry to 165° F and poultry parts to 180° F. Reheat pre-cooked meats until steaming hot.

When taking foods off the grill, don't put the cooked items on the same platter which held the raw meat. Raw meat juices can contain bacteria that could cross-contaminate safely cooked foods.

Do not partially grill extra hamburgers to use later. Once you begin cooking hamburgers by any method, cook them until completely done to assure that bacteria are destroyed.

Keeping Leftovers Safe

Place leftover foods in the cooler promptly after grilling or serving. Any left outside for more than an hour should be discarded.

For the return trip, the cooler should again travel in the air-conditioned part of the car. If you were gone not more than 4 or 5 hours and your perishables were kept on ice except when cooked and served, you should be able to use the leftovers.

Check the cooler when you get home. If there is still ice in the cooler and the food is "refrigerator cool" to the touch, the leftovers should be safe to eat.

For Further Information

FSIS Food Safety Education and Communications Staff
Meat and Poultry Hotline:
1-800-535-4555 (Tollfree Nationwide)
(202) 720-3333 (Washington, DC area)
1-800-256-7072 (TDD/TTY)

For additional food safety information about meat, poultry, or eggs, call the toll-free USDA Meat and Poultry Hotline at 1 (800) 535-4555; Washington, D.C., call (202) 720-3333; TTY: 1 (800) 256-7072. It is staffed by home economists, dietitians, and food technologists from 10 a.m. to 4 p.m. Eastern time, year round. An extensive selection of food safety recordings can be heard 24 hours a day using a touch-tone phone.

Information is also available from the FSIS Web site: http://www.fsis.usda.gov/.

Chapter 41

Advice for Packing Safe School Lunches

School bells are tolling around the country as students begin a new school year. Although millions buy lunch at school cafeterias, millions more bring their lunch in the familiar paper bag or lunch box.

"Now is the time for students to not only learn their ABC's, but also food safety basics when bringing lunch to school," says Bessie Berry, Manager of the U.S. Department of Agriculture's nationwide, toll-free Meat and Poultry Hotline. "Safe bag lunches are as important as learning math and science. In fact, food safety is a science."

Berry said that by following some simple food safety rules, students can avoid getting sick from a lunch that was not handled properly. Here are some basic tips for carrying a safe lunch to school:

Keep Foods Clean

Keep everything clean when packing the lunch. That not only goes for the food, but also food preparation surfaces, hands and utensils. Use hot, soapy water. Keep family pets away from kitchen counters. "Wash your hands before you prepare or eat food," Berry explains.

Keep Cold Foods Cold

The best way to keep food cold is with an insulated lunch box. When packing lunches, include either freezer gel packs widely available in

An undated fact sheet produced by the Food Safety and Inspection Service; United States Department of Agriculture, Washington, D.C. 20250-3700.

stores or cold food items such as fruit, or small frozen juice packs. Nestle perishable meat, poultry or egg sandwiches between these cold items. Sandwiches can also be made ahead of time and kept refrigerated or frozen before placing in the lunch box.

Freezer gel packs will hold cold foods until lunchtime, but generally will not work for all-day storage. "Any perishable leftovers after lunch should be discarded and not brought home," Berry advises.

Instead of the insulated lunch box, can brown paper bags or plastic lunch bags be used to store cold foods? "These are OK, but do not work as well as insulated lunch boxes because the bags tend to become soggy and do not retain the cold as well," Berry explains. "If you must use paper or plastic lunch bags, create layers by double bagging to help insulate the food." Also, control the environment where the lunch bag or box is kept at school to help keep foods cold. Keep out of direct sunlight and away from radiators or other heat sources.

Keep Hot Foods Hot

Foods like soup, chili and stew need to stay hot. Use an insulated bottle stored in an insulated lunch box. Fill the bottle with boiling water, let stand for a few minutes, empty, and then put in the piping hot food. Keep the insulated bottle closed until lunch to keep the food hot.

For More Information

For more information on packing safe lunches for school (and yes, work, too!) call the toll-free nationwide Meat and Poultry Hotline at 1-800-535-4555. In the Washington, D.C. area, the number is 202-720-3333.

The Hotline is open Monday through Friday from 10 a.m. to 4 p.m., Eastern Time, year-round. Also, an extensive selection of timely food safety recordings are available 24 hours a day, every day, by using a touch-tone phone and the "user-friendly" menu which prompts callers.

In addition, helpful food safety information is now available on the Internet. Simply call up the USDA Food Safety and Inspection Service Home Page at home or school. The address is http://www.usda.gov/fsis. The Home Page is an electronic avenue by which students and others can "click" icons to a wealth of food safety and handling subjects.

For Further Information, Contact:

FSIS Food Safety Education and Communications Staff
Meat and Poultry Hotline
Phone: 1-800-535-4555

Chapter 42

Keep Your Baby Safe

Eat Hard Cheeses Instead of Soft Cheeses During Pregnancy

As a pregnant woman, eating for two, you should be aware that certain soft cheeses can become contaminated with bacteria called *Listeria*. If you become sick from *Listeria*, the baby you're carrying could get sick or die. To protect your unborn baby, eat hard cheeses instead of soft cheeses while you are pregnant.

Soft cheeses that can easily become contaminated include:

- Mexican-Style Soft Cheeses
  - queso blanco   queso de crema
  - queso fresco   asadero
  - queso de hoja

- Other Soft Cheeses
  - feta (goat cheese)
  - brie
  - Camembert
  - blue-veined cheeses, like Roquefort

Listeria can also contaminate other foods. Contaminated food may not look, smell or taste different from uncontaminated food.

FDA Brochure: June 1996; Updated July 1997; U. S. Food and Drug Administration, Center for Food Safety and Applied Nutrition.

233

Symptoms of infection can develop from 2 to 30 days after you eat contaminated food. If the infection spreads to your unborn baby, you could start early labor. Tell your doctor right away if you get any of these symptoms:

- fever and chills, or other flu-like symptoms
- headache
- nausea
- vomiting

Although *Listeria* bacteria are killed with thorough cooking, these "tough bugs" can grow in the refrigerator and survive in the freezer. To prevent infection, take these precautions:

- Use hard cheeses, like cheddar, instead of soft cheeses during pregnancy. If you do use soft cheeses during pregnancy, cook them until they are boiling (bubbling).

- Use only pasteurized dairy products. It will state "pasteurized" on the label.

- If you do use hard cheeses made from unpasteurized milk, use only those marked "aged 60 days" (or longer).

- Eat only thoroughly cooked meat, poultry or seafood.

- Thoroughly reheat all meats purchased at deli counters, including cured meats like salami, before eating them.

- Wash all fruits and vegetables with water.

- Follow label instructions on products that must be refrigerated or that have a "use by" date.

- Keep the inside of the refrigerator, counter tops, and utensils clean.

- After handling raw foods, wash your hands with warm soapy water, and wash the utensil you used with hot soapy water before using them again.

Do you have any questions about *Listeria*? Call (1-800) FDA-4010.

Department of Health and Human Services
Food and Drug Administration (HFI-40)
5600 Fishers Lane, Rockville, MD 20857
DHHS Publication No. (FDA) 96-2304S

Part Four

The Food Handler's Role in Food Safety

Chapter 43

A Menu of Modern Safety Standards

The carefully cleaned vegetables in the grocery salad bar, the fully-cooked hamburgers at the neighborhood fast-food restaurant, the fresh cold milk on the lunch tray at the nursing home—these foods are all prepared by people who pay attention to details. If they were not so careful, it's possible they could unknowingly cause someone to get sick from any one of the many illnesses that could be spread through food. And in this day of emerging dangerous strains of bacteria, attention to detail is especially important.

Most of the heightened awareness and the food safety routines required of people who prepare and serve food directly to consumers originate with the Food and Drug Administration's *Food Code*. The *Food Code*, revised in 1998 to combine three documents into one, recommends new procedures for food establishment workers based on the latest scientific thinking on how to prevent foodborne disease.

Included are new recommendations for cooking times and temperatures to kill dangerous bacteria that could be present in food, and for holding times and temperatures to slow or prevent growth. And, for the first time, the *Code* will give instructions for the proper use of food additives. Also included are basics, such as cleaning hands, employee health, cleaning food, preparation and serving areas, and managers' responsibilities.

The *Food Code* is neither federal law nor regulation. Rather, it is offered as model legislation to more than 85 state and territorial agencies and 3,000 local regulatory departments that license and inspect

FDA Consumer, April 1994, U.S. Food and Drug Administration.

the more than 1 million establishments in the United States offering food directly to consumers.

State and local jurisdictions use the code to develop or update their own food rules. Officials with experience using older editions of food codes helped with the 1998 revision. The 1998 Food Code is the 17th edition. The first was published in 1934.

"The code gives the public health community the information it needs to speak with one voice about what's important for food safety and what it expects of food establishment operators," says Art Banks of FDA's retail food protection branch and chief architect of the document.

Federal agencies that direct their own food services, such as the U.S. Interior Department's Park Service and the Department of Defense, apply *Food Code* guidelines directly to their operations. The Navajo Nation has also adopted earlier editions of the *Food Code* for use in their food establishments.

Code Changes

"The *Food Code* has changed a great deal over the years," says Banks, "because food operations at the retail level have changed significantly." Previously, the code was three separate documents—one each for food service (last published in 1976), food vending (1978), and food stores (1982). The 1993 edition combined the three into one document and has been updated every two years. Banks calls the new combined edition a "full tool box" that covers all categories food operations are likely to encounter.

Combining the codes was necessary, he says, because "the lines have blurred" that distinguish the types of services offered by retail food operations. For example, some restaurants now sell featured ingredients from their own entrées, such as barbecue sauces and bakery items, as groceries.

Grocery stores have self-service salad bars and ready-to-eat entrées in their delicatessens. Although enthusiasm for self-serve bulk foods is fading somewhat, many stores still offer them. Convenience stores often sell store-prepared fast food items such as hot dogs, pizzas, and breakfast entrées. And many food store and food service operations have vending machines.

In addition, restaurants and grocers are now using new ingredients and preparing foods in ways that were not envisioned when previous codes were written. "Today, consumers' wants and needs go beyond the traditional," Banks says. "Cooks don't always use the common spices you find in most kitchens, and their equipment is much more sophisticated." These expanded cooking styles and procedures—house-smoked sausage, for example—mean added responsibilities for food service managers and restaurant inspectors.

"Today's restaurant inspectors deal with federally regulated food additives, such as sulfites," continues Banks. Sulfites are sulfur-based preservatives legally used in many foods, including most bottled lemon juice and some frozen shrimp. Applied directly to produce, such as in salad bars, sulfites maintain color and perk up crispness. But sulfites can cause life-threatening reactions in people who are sulfite-sensitive, so federal law prohibits food service establishments from using them on fresh produce (see "A Fresh Look at Food Preservatives" in the October 1993 *FDA Consumer*). This is part of the *Food Code* advice on food additives.

As food processing technology progresses, food service operations increasingly depend on ready-to-serve foods that are sometimes used "as is" or combined with other ingredients. The new *Food Code* includes special handling requirements for ready-to-eat foods because of their potential to spoil or to carry harmful food-borne organisms. "It used to be that a cook prepared coleslaw from locally purchased cabbage," says Banks. "These days, that coleslaw might be prepared at a food processing plant several states away, or a pre-prepared entrée could arrive vacuum-packed in plastic pouches," explains Banks.

Controlling Bad Bugs

"One of the problems we have today is the emergence of adaptive organisms-especially virulent pathogens transmitted through food that survive changing conditions," Banks says. "For example," he explains, "cooking hamburgers to a temperature of 140° Fahrenheit used to be sufficient to kill most harmful organisms. But in order to kill *Escherichia coli* 0 1 57:H7, a bacterial strain of emerging importance that has caused death in young children, hamburger must now be cooked to 155° F and maintained at that temperature for at least 15 seconds." (Food service establishments usually have equipment to precisely measure cooking temperatures. However, since most homes do not, FDA and the U.S. Department of Agriculture recommend, for assurance of safety, that consumers cook ground meat to the higher temperature of 160° F. (See "How to Outsmart a Dangerous *E. Coli* Strain" in the January-February 1994 FDA Consumer.)

Another problem is *Salmonella enteritidis*. In the past, cracked and dirty eggs were a common source of illness caused by *Salmonella*.

Improvements in shell egg production, cleaning and packaging have greatly reduced the problem. "The concern now," says Banks, "is that one of the *Salmonella* strains that causes most human infections, *Salmonella enteritidis*, in some cases may be carried inside the egg and transmitted by infected hens before the shell is formed."

Another *Salmonella* strain has also been found on cut melons, such as those served in salad bars. Food safety experts believe this type of contamination probably stems from not properly washing the melon before cutting, transferring bacteria still on its surface from harvest to the melon's inside. It's also possible that bacteria are transmitted from improperly washed hands or the knife used to cut the melon.

"Thorough cooking and proper preparation can eliminate foodborne problems such as *E. coli* 0 157: H7 or *Salmonella* that could occur upstream, before food reaches the retail level," says Banks. "But no one wants a hamburger that resembles a hockey puck, or eggs cooked to the consistency of cardboard," he says.

To ensure that food is palatable as well as safely cooked, the new *Food Code* shows different cooking times, temperatures, and holding times for foods that have the potential to cause illness. For example, safe cooking times and temperatures sometimes differ for the same food, depending on how it's prepared. A beef roast has different cooking and holding requirements than ground beef, and eggs broken from the shell and prepared for immediate serving may be cooked differently than eggs that have been pooled for use during the breakfast serving time. There are also time and temperature recommendations for poultry and game animals, corned beef, and other meat and fish products such as stuffed poultry, meat, fish, and pasta, and stuffing that contains meat, fish or poultry.

"It's impossible for cooks to remember all those numbers without some ready reference," says Banks.

Working with Watchers

"FDA can't watch everything," says Banks. "There are well over a million retail food establishments in the United States in any number of localities and types of food preparation and services. That's where local inspectors and licensing agencies take on the job of food safety surveillance," he says.

Not every locality uses the *Food Code* in the same manner. For instance, Dan Sowards, a Texas Department of Health official, says his state will not adopt the entire *Food Code*, but will use it to revise and amend the Texas food code, which addresses food protection issues that are specific to the region. Sowards finds particularly useful certain sanitation provisions. "The revised code deals very efficiently with employee hygiene and the responsibilities of management for training employees in that area."

Both government and the food industry share the responsibility for food safety. The Food Code, with its overlapping safeguards to prevent foodborne illness, is provided to help ensure that consumers will be able to eat out or shop for food with confidence.

How Clean Is Clean?

How clean is clean enough for the hands of food service workers?

"A 20-second scrub for hands and exposed parts of the arms with soap, then a rinse with clear water, says Arthur Banks, FDA's retail food protection branch chief. "And if a worker has used the toilet, that worker must use a nail brush with soap to clean fingertips and under fingernails. Then the scrub with soap alone is repeated for another 20 seconds. That's much more time than most people spend washing their hands," Banks says.

Workers must wear single-use plastic gloves and use tongs or "deli" paper tissues or other means to avoid bare-hand contact with ready-to-eat foods that will not be further cooked.

Hands need to be washed:

- after touching bare human body parts

- after using the toilet

- after handling support animals, such as guard or seeing-eye dogs

- after coughing or sneezing (even when using a tissue), using tobacco, eating, or drinking

- after handling soiled equipment or utensils

- immediately before and during food preparation as often as necessary to remove soil and to prevent cross-contamination when changing tasks, such as changing from raw meat to raw produce

- during food preparation when switching between raw foods and ready-to-eat foods.

FDA says that bar soaps are acceptable for hand washing. For years, there has been concern that bar soaps might be capable of becoming contaminated with and transmitting infectious organisms. Some have argued that liquid or powdered soap from individual-portion dispensers might therefore be the best choice for hand washing.

The scientific data on this subject are inconclusive. Studies by two soap manufacturers show no bacterial transmission through bar soap use, but studies by university researchers refute this.

Robert Haley, M.D., University of Texas, formerly of the national Centers for Disease Control and Prevention, is quoted in a February 1984 article in the industry publication *Soap / Cosmetics / Chemical Specialties* as saying, "more research is necessary before any connection between contaminated soap bars and transmission of sickness can be established. " The article also pointed out that liquid soap has occasionally been found to be contaminated with disease-causing microorganisms that could be transmitted at the hand contact surface of the dispensers.

Chapter 44

The Impact of Consumer Demands and Trends on Food Processing

In the United States, consumer demand for new foods and changes in eating habits and food safety risks are affecting the food processing industry. The population is becoming older on average; moreover, consumers want fresh and minimally processed foods without synthetic chemical preservatives. To address the need for safer food and compete for consumer acceptance, manufacturers are exploring new food processing and preservation methods.

Fresh, Preservative-Free Foods That Promote Health

Food industry marketers perceive that consumers want foods that are convenient; fresh (less-processed and less-packaged); all natural—with no preservatives (a so-called "clean label"); without a perceived negative (i.e., foods without high fat, high salt, and high sugar); and healthy. The industry perception is that consumers want foods that not only cause no harm but also remedy ailments from heart disease, osteoporosis, and fatigue to memory loss. Categories of foods that promote health are fortified foods, performance-enhancing food additives, probiotics, and prebiotics.

Food fortification is an old process. Milk (with vitamins A and D), bread (with iron and niacin), or salt (with iodine) have long been fortified to replace nutrients thought to be lost during processing. Newer foods fortified with nutrients needed by the body to stave off the progression of diseases associated with aging or enhance physical

© Nestlé USA, Inc., Glendale, California, USA; reprinted with permission.

performance attract the consumer's attention and sell well in today's marketplace. For example, marketers are promoting all sorts of foods fortified with calcium to women concerned about osteoporosis. Performance-enhancing foods are popular. Such foods range from beverages to replace electrolytes and prolong physical endurance to amino acids and fatty acids to improve alertness and memory. Probiotics and prebiotics are two paths to the same result. Research studies suggest that a desirable intestinal microflora causes the host to be less susceptible to intestinal pathogens. Probiotics create this desirable state by incorporating the microorganism directly into the food, either as a stable culture or as part of food fermentation. This process is costly, and the microorganisms often do not survive well in the food. Thus, manufacturers must add 10 to 100 times the needed number of microorganisms to account for a loss of viability during the product's normal shelf life. Prebiotics overcomes the limitations of probiotics by adding specific nutrients, usually a particular carbohydrate, to the food. When ingested as part of the diet, these specific nutrients "select" for a beneficial microflora in the intestinal tract.

Food Processing and Food Product Development

The consumer's quest for health is having a great impact on the food processor. Compared with the marketplace of 25 years ago, today's marketplace has more perishable products, including fruits and vegetables, and more innovative packaging. In addition, consumer aversion to traditional chemical preservatives has left food processors with less flexibility in choosing preservation methods. To find a technologic edge in the marketplace, food processors are exploring new processing and preservation technologies. Some of these technologies include ohmic heating, high-pressure, pulsed electric field, bright light, and aseptic processing. Ohmic heating involves passing an electric current through the food to create heat due to electrical resistance within the food. With ohmic heating, food particles heat at the same rate as the carrier medium or sauce. Ohmic heating can enhance food quality by limiting heat damage to the sauce and food particles. High-pressure processing uses very high pressure, often thousands of atmospheres, to pasteurize foods without heat. This technology is ideal for heat-sensitive foods, but some enzymes are difficult to inactivate with high-pressure processing. Pulsed electric field processing uses a very strong pulsed electric current to disrupt microbial cells and pasteurize foods with little or no heating. Bright light processing uses an intense white light to kill bacteria on the surface of foods; this light does not penetrate deeply into foods and can only be used for surface pasteurization.

Aseptic processing dates back to at least the mid-1940s but has yet to realize its full potential. The most widely used of these new technologies, aseptic processing involves sterilizing a food product in a continuous process through a heat exchanger and then filling that food in an aseptic filler. The aseptic filler is a highly specialized piece of equipment designed to sterilize the packaging material, fill the sterile product into its container in a sterile environment, and then seal the package.

Food processors have also explored novel food preservation systems. An ideal food preservative would come from a natural source and preserve food without being labeled a synthetic chemical preservative. Such preservatives include bacteriocins, dimethyl dicarbonate (Velcorin), competitive microbial inhibition, controlled and modified atmospheres, and irradiation. Bacteriocins are not new; however, like nisin, they are now being used to extend shelf life and enhance the safety of a variety of food products. The use of bacteriocins is likely to be expanded in the future. Dimethyl dicarbonate, a relatively new preservative used in beverages such as wine, tea, and juices, is particularly effective in preventing spoilage caused by yeasts. Competitive microbial inhibition relies on the fact that many harmless bacteria, notably lactic acid bacteria, can inhibit the growth of both spoilage bacteria and pathogens. Inhibitory strains of lactic acid bacteria can be selected for use in dairy cultures or be added to refrigerated foods to extend shelf life and enhance safety. Modified and controlled atmosphere packaging are already widely used by the food industry. They have the potential for even wider use, particularly with fresh fruits and vegetables sold at retail. These methods rely on inhibiting microbial growth by excluding oxygen or by inhibitory concentrations of carbon dioxide. Carefully selected gas mixtures can also delay the ripening of certain fruits and vegetables and extend the shelf life of fresh meats. Finally, irradiation, also not a new technology, is poised for widespread use to enhance the safety and shelf life of many foods. With proper controls, irradiation could be a valuable means of reducing Salmonella contamination of poultry and *Escherichia coli* O157:H7 contamination of ground beef.

A Scientist's View of Consumer Trends

One of the most obvious consumer trends is a dramatic increase in the consumption of fresh foods, particularly fruits and vegetables.

This increase is the result of the well-publicized value of a high-fiber diet and betacarotenes as an aid in preventing colon cancer. The number of meals eaten away from home has increased dramatically. The trend toward dining outside the home is likely rooted in lifestyle changes such as households with two working parents. The number of home-delivered meals, the ultimate convenience food, has also increased, even though the most popular foods consumed today (pizza and hamburgers) are generally the same as those of 20 years ago. This indicates that the types of foods consumed do not change rapidly, but the way these foods are consumed has changed. Finally, the population is getting older on average. Aging may not be a consumer trend, but it has a profound effect on food safety considerations. An older population means a more susceptible population.

New food processing and preservation technologies and wider applications of older technologies have, for the most part, had little impact on most processed foods. Adoption of new technologies will likely continue at a slow pace. Consumers consistently buy foods on the basis of value and taste, not processing technology. Technologies that add value will be the first to gain consumer acceptance. The demand for convenience foods will probably increase. Demands on our time are increasing, and we have less time to spend on food preparation, and more meals will be eaten away from home, in part because of convenience but also because of a trend for new tastes and variety in the diet. Finally, the trend toward foods that claim to enhance performance, rooted in an aging population's need for better health during longer life-spans, will continue. With increased demand, the pressure on the food industry for better processing and preservation methods will also increase and may result in safer food.

— by Don L. Zink

Nestlé USA, Inc. 800 N. Brand Blvd., Glendale, CA 91203, USA; fax: 818-549-6908; e-mail: donald.zink@us.nestle.com.

Chapter 45

Food Product Dating

"Sell by Feb 14" is a type of information you might find on a meat or poultry product. Are dates required on food products? Does it mean the product will be unsafe to use after that date? Here is some background information which answers these and other questions about product dating.

What is Dating?

"Open Dating" (use of a calendar date as opposed to a code) on a food product is a date stamped on a product's package to help the store determine how long to display the product for sale. It can also help the purchaser to know the time limit to purchase or use the product at its best quality. It is not a safety date.

Is Dating Required by Federal Law?

Except for infant formula and some baby food (see below), product dating is not required by Federal regulations. However, if a calendar date is used, it must express both the month and day of the month (and the year, in the case of shelf-stable and frozen products). If a calendar date is shown, immediately adjacent to the date must be a phrase explaining the meaning of that date such as "sell by" or "use before."

Consumer Education and Information, March 1995; Food Safety and Inspection Service United States Department of Agriculture; Washington, D.C. 20250-3700.

There is no uniform or universally accepted system used for food dating in the United States. Although dating of some foods is required by more than 20 states, there are areas of the country where much of the food supply has some type of open date and other areas where almost no food is dated.

What Types of Food Are Dated?

Open dating is found primarily on perishable foods such as meat, poultry, eggs and dairy products. "Closed" or "coded" dating might appear on shelf-stable products such as cans and boxes of food.

Types of Dates

- A "Sell-By" date tells the store how long to display the product for sale. You should buy the product before the date expires.

- A "Best if Used By (or Before)" date is recommended for best flavor or quality. It is not a purchase or safety date.

- A "Use-By" date is the last date recommended for the use of the product while at peak quality. The date has been determined by the manufacturer of the product.

- "Closed or coded dates" are packing numbers for use by the manufacturer.

Safety After Date Expires

Except for "use-by" dates, product dates don't always refer to home storage and use after purchase. But even if the date expires during home storage, a product should be safe, wholesome and of good quality—if handled properly and kept at 40° F or below. See the accompanying refrigerator charts for storage times of dated products.

Foods can develop an off odor, flavor or appearance due to spoilage bacteria. If a food has developed such characteristics, you should not use it for quality reasons.

If foods are mishandled, however, foodborne bacteria can grow and cause foodborne illness—before or after the date on the package. For example, if hot dogs are taken to a picnic and left out several hours, they wouldn't be safe if used thereafter, even if the date hasn't expired.

Other examples of potential mishandling are products that have been: defrosted at room temperature more than two hours; cross contaminated;

or handled by people who don't use proper sanitary practices. Make sure to follow the handling and preparation instructions on the label to ensure top quality and safety.

Can a Retailer Change Dates?

A retailer may legally sell fresh or processed meat and poultry products beyond the expiration date on the package as long as the product is wholesome.

It is also legal for a retailer to change a date on wholesome fresh meat that has been cut up and wrapped in the meat department of the supermarket.

However, it is not legal to modify a label on a product packaged under federal inspection. If a product has an expired date and the food remains wholesome, the product may continue to be offered for sale but the expired date cannot be altered, changed or covered up by a new date.

A special case is infant formula and some baby food. Do not buy or use it past the date and do not purchase it if the date has been changed.

Dating Formula and Baby Food

Federal regulations require a use-by date on the product label of infant formula and the varieties of baby food under FDA inspection. If consumed by that date, the formula or food must contain not less than the quantity of each nutrient as described on the label. Formula must maintain an acceptable quality to pass through an ordinary bottle nipple. If stored too long, formula can separate and clog the nipple.

Dating of baby food is for quality as well as for nutrient retention. Just as you might not want to eat stale potato chips, you wouldn't want to feed your baby meat or other foods that have an off flavor or texture.

The use-by date is selected by the manufacturer, packer or distributor of the product on the basis of product analysis throughout its shelf life; tests; or other information. It is also based on the conditions of handling, storage, preparation and use printed on the label. Do not buy or use baby formula or baby food after its use-by date.

What Do Can Codes Mean?

Cans must exhibit a packing code to enable tracking of the product in interstate commerce. This enables manufacturers to rotate their stock as well as to locate their products in the event of a recall.

These codes, which appear as a series of letters and/or numbers, might refer to the date or time of manufacture. They aren't meant for the consumer to interpret as "use-by" dates. There is no book which tells how to translate the codes into dates.

Cans may also display "open" or calendar dates. Usually these are "best if used by" dates for peak quality.

In general, high-acid canned foods such as tomatoes, grapefruit and pineapple can be stored on the shelf 12 to 18 months; low-acid canned foods such as meat, poultry, fish and most vegetables will keep 2 to 5 years—if the can remains in good condition and has been stored in a cool, clean, dry place.

Dates on Egg Cartons

If the egg carton has an expiration date printed on it, such as "EXP May 1," be sure that the date has not passed when the eggs are purchased. That is the last day the store may sell the eggs as fresh.

On eggs which have a Federal grademark, such as Grade AA, the date cannot be more than 30 days from the date the eggs were packed into the carton.

As long as you purchase a carton of eggs before the date expires, you should be able to use all the eggs safely in three to five weeks after the date you purchase them.

UPC or Bar Codes

Universal Product Codes appear on packages as black lines of varying widths above a series of numbers. They are not required by regulation but manufacturers print them on most product labels because scanners at supermarkets can "read" them quickly to record the price at checkout.

Bar codes are used by stores and manufacturers for inventory purposes and marketing information. When read by a computer, they can reveal such specific information as the manufacturer's name, product name, size of product and price. The numbers are not used to identify recalled products.

Storage Times

Since product dates aren't a guide for safe use of a product, how long can the consumer store the food and still use it at top quality? Follow these tips:

- Purchase the product before the date expires.

- If perishable, take the food home immediately after purchase and refrigerate it promptly. Freeze it if you can't use it within times recommended on chart.

- Once a perishable product is frozen, it doesn't matter if the date expires because foods kept frozen continuously are safe indefinitely.

- Follow handling recommendations on product.

- Consult the following storage chart.

- Refrigerator home storage (at 40° F or below) of fresh or uncooked products.

- If product has a "Use-By Date," follow that date.

If product has a "Sell-By Date" or no date, cook or freeze the product by the times shown in Table 45.1.

Table 45.1. Storage Tips: If product has a "Sell-By Date" or no date, cook or freeze the product by the times shown.

Product	Storage Times After Purchase
Poultry	1 or 2 days
Beef, Veal, Pork and Lamb	3 to 5 days
Ground Meat and Ground Poultry	1 or 2 days
Fresh Variety Meats (Liver, Tongue, Brain, Kidneys, Heart, Chitterlings)	1 or 2 days
Cured Ham, Cook Before-Eating	5 to 7 days
Sausage from Pork, Beef or Turkey, Uncooked	1 or 2 days
Eggs	3 to 5 weeks

Refrigerator Home Storage (40° F or below) of Processed Products Sealed at Plant

If product has a "Use-By Date," follow that date.

If product has a "Sell-By Date" or no date, cook or freeze the product by the times in Table 45.2.

Table 46.5. Processed Products Sealed at Plant: If product has a "Sell-By Date" or no date, cook or freeze the product by the times.

Processed Product	Unopened, After Purchase	After Opening
Cooked Poultry	3 to 4 days	3 to 4 days
Cooked Sausage	3 to 4 days	3 to 4 days
Sausage, Hard/Dry, shelf-stable	6 weeks/pantry	3 weeks
Corned Beef, uncooked, in pouch with pickling juices	5 to 7 days	3 to 4 days
Vacuum-packed Dinners, Commercial Brand with USDA seal	2 weeks	3 to 4 days
Bacon	2 weeks	7 days
Hotdogs	2 weeks (but no longer than 1 week after a "sell-by" date)	7 days
Lunch Meats	2 weeks (but no longer than 1 week after a "sell-by" date)	3 to 5 days
Ham, fully cooked	7 days	slices, 3 days; whole, 7 days
Ham, canned, labeled "keep refrigerated"	9 months	3 to 4 days
Ham, canned, shelf stable	2 years/pantry	3 to 5 days
Canned Meat and Poultry, shelf stable	2 to 5 years/pantry	3 to 4 days

For additional food safety information about meat, poultry or eggs, call the toll-free USDA Meat and Poultry Hotline at 1 (800) 535-4555. It is staffed by home economists from 10 a.m. to 4 p.m. ET year round. An extensive selection of food safety recordings can be heard 24 hours a day using a touch-tone phone.

For Further Information Contact:

FSIS Food Safety Education and Communications Staff
Meat and Poultry Hotline:
1-800-535-4555 (Tollfree Nationwide)

Chapter 46

Foodborne Illnesses in the Child Care Setting

Food safety and sanitation are important aspects of providing healthy food for children. Improper food preparation, handling, or storage can quickly result in food being contaminated with germs that may lead to illness such as hepatitis A or diarrheal diseases if the contaminated food is eaten. Contact your local health department to obtain the local regulations and standards for food safety and sanitation and to ask about the availability of a food handler course in your area.

Understanding and following a few basic principles can help prevent food spoilage and transmission of infections. To prevent foodborne infections:

- Keep food at safe serving and storage temperatures at all times to prevent spoiling and the risk of transmitting disease. Food should be kept at 40°F or colder or at 140°F or warmer. The range between 40°F and 140°F is considered the "danger zone" because within this range bacteria grow most easily. Leftovers, including hot foods such as soups or sauces, should be refrigerated immediately and should not be left to cool at room temperature. Using shallow pans or bowls will facilitate rapid cooling. Frozen foods should be thawed in the refrigerator, not on counter tops, or in the sink with cold water, not hot or warm water.

An undated fact sheet produced by the Centers for Disease Control and Prevention.

- Use only approved food preparation equipment, dishes, and utensils. Check local childcare licensing regulations. Only use cutting boards that can be disinfected (made of nonporous materials such as glass, formica, or plastic), and use separate boards for ready-to-eat foods (including foods to be eaten raw) and for foods which are to be cooked, such as meats.

- Use proper handwashing techniques. Proper handwashing is important for everyone in a child-care setting, but is especially necessary for food handlers to prevent the spread of infections or contamination of the food.

- Don't handle food if you change diapers. In a large childcare setting, food handlers should not change diapers and should avoid other types of contact that may contaminate their hands with infectious secretions. This may not be practical in a small childcare setting in which the provider must also prepare the food. In this case, proper handwashing is essential.

- Don't prepare or serve food if you have diarrhea, unusually loose stools, or any other gastrointestinal symptoms of an illness, or if you have infected skin sores or injuries, or open cuts. Small, uninfected cuts may be covered with nonporous, latex gloves.

- Supervise meal and snack times to make sure children do not share plates, utensils, or food that is not individually wrapped.

- Eating utensils that are dropped on the floor should be washed with soap and water before using.

- Discard food that is dropped on the floor and remove leftovers from the eating area after each snack or meal.

- Clean, sanitize, and properly store food service equipment and supplies. Use only utensils and dishes that have been washed in a dishwasher or, if washed by hand, with sanitizers and disinfectants approved for this use. Otherwise, use disposable, single-use articles that are discarded after each use.

- Clean and sanitize after each use tabletops on which food is served.

- Only accept expressed breast milk that is fresh and properly labeled with the child's name. Expressed breast milk to be used during the current shift should accompany the child that day. Don't store breast milk at the facility overnight. Send any unused expressed breast milk home with the child that day. NEVER feed a child breast milk unless it is labeled with that child's name.

- Except for an individual child's lunch, only accept food that is commercially prepared to be brought into the childcare setting. Numerous institutional outbreaks of gastrointestinal illness, including infectious hepatitis, have been linked to consumption of home-prepared foods. Food brought into the childcare setting to celebrate birthdays, holidays, or other special occasions should be obtained from commercial sources approved and inspected by the local health authority.

- Each individual child's lunch brought from home should be clearly labeled with the child's name, the date, and the type of food it is. It should be stored at an appropriate temperature until it is eaten. Food brought from a child's home should not be fed to another child.

- Raw eggs can be contaminated with Salmonella. No foods containing raw eggs should be served, including homemade ice cream made with raw eggs.

Chapter 47

In Day-Care Centers, Cleanliness Is a Must

Day-care centers have become a way of life in America. More than half of all mothers of children too young to care for themselves hold jobs outside the home. For them—indeed for millions of American families—day-care centers provide a service that is a necessity. If both parents work, a solo parent caring for a child must work, or other family support systems are inadequate, child day care answers a critical need. Unfortunately, though, it often provides something else—a focal point for certain kinds of infectious diseases that can all to easily spread not only to others in the day-care center, but far and wide into the community.

The problem involves illnesses, particularly enteric (small intestine) infections, that usually show themselves as diarrhea and other disturbances in the gastrointestinal tract.

Enteric illnesses are commonly associated with "food poisoning." But in the nation's day-care centers, tainted food is often not the culprit. Rather, the illnesses most often result from fecal contamination because staff and children fail to follow the dictates of ordinary common sense about things like hand washing and cleanliness.

The major contributors to the spread of enteric diseases—person-to-person contact, water and food—are interrelated and part of a persistent cycle. Attacking one part of the problem will have little effect. What's needed is a concerted effort directed at all sources of transmission of enteric pathogens.

FDA Consumer, August 1989, updated December 1995, U. S. Food and Drug Administration.

Studies show that children under 3 who are cared for in day-care centers are more subject to diarrheal attacks than other youngsters. Likewise, day-care center workers and families of these young day-care children seem to suffer more bouts of diarrhea. L.K. Pickering, M.D., a professor of pediatrics at the University of Texas, noted in an editorial in the *American Journal of Public Health* that diarrhea was 30 percent more common in day-care children than in children cared for at home.

Another study found that day-care children under 3 had diarrhea twice as often as children remaining at home. A study reported in the September 1988 journal *Pediatrics* found an average of 3.8 diarrhea outbreaks per child per year in day-care centers in Houston, Texas. Similar findings have been reported from cities throughout the United States.

A recent family survey by Pickering and his colleagues showed that the average head of household or spouse lost 13 workdays because of illness in his or her day-care-center child; just under five of those lost days were due to diarrheal disease.

The spread of enteric illnesses to family members is documented in several surveys, one of which found that 10 of 56 family members of ill children were afflicted but only 1 of 45 family members of well children developed the illness. The episodes can be quite severe. One study reported a median duration of 12 days, while another noted that episodes lasted as long as six weeks. Hospitalizations were not all that infrequent.

The cause of these infections is usually some well-known pathogen such as the hepatitis A virus, rotavirus, *Giardia, E. coli, Cryptosporidium, Shigella,* or *Campytobacter.*

The human gut, including that of small children, normally contains many of the pathogenic bacteria and viruses that can cause diarrhea, but the body's natural defenses usually keep them well under control. More important, these potentially dangerous organisms don't ordinarily get spread around. But fecal contamination can be a prime source of disease in centers that care for children under 3—those still in diapers and still being toilet trained. Hands, toys, diaper-changing areas, and just about everything else can be contaminated with fecal matter. Children and adults who touch these contaminated objects and then put their fingers to their mouths are prime candidates for disease.

A microbiologist in FDA's Center for Food Safety and Applied Nutrition, writing in the January/February 1989 issue of the *Journal of Environmental Health*, cautioned that diarrhea may not be the only consequence of fecal contamination in day-care centers. Noting that children generally have symptoms far longer than adults do, he commented that diarrhea persisting a week or more can lead to nutrient losses and can also compromise the immune system. Further, in an important reminder that all of us should heed, he pointed out that both a form of arthritis and certain neuromuscular disorders have been associated with bacteria that cause diarrhea. And he reported the disquieting fact that some of the strains of pathogens causing outbreaks of diarrheal disease are extremely resistant to commonly used disinfectants.

Nevertheless, there are things day-care centers can do to minimize the danger of infection caused by fecal contamination. Preventive measures include:

- Hand washing. As simple as it may seem, hand washing is, as Professor Pickering says, "the single most preventive measure in the day-care center." Indeed, one study showed that outbreaks could be cut in half simply by requiring staff and children to wash their hands after diaper changes and bowel movements;

- Providing separate diaper-changing areas, preferably with disposable cover sheets and smooth, nonabsorbent, easily cleaned surfaces;

- Cleaning and disinfecting the diapering area after each use;

- Keeping younger children—especially those in diapers—separate from older children during the day;

- Keeping children with diarrhea at home;

- Segregating children whose diarrhea has stopped but who may still be carriers;

- Providing staff education on preventive measures and regular follow-ups to be sure the measures are being taken.

The U.S. Centers for Disease Control describes proper hand washing as follows:

- Use soap and running water.

- Rub your hands vigorously as you wash them.

- Wash all surfaces (including backs of hands, wrists, between fingers, and under fingernails).

- Rinse well and leave the water running.

- Dry hands with a single-use towel.

- Turn off water using a paper towel covering freshly washed hands.

Day-care staff members should wash their hands when they start work, before preparing or serving food, after diapering a child or wiping his nose or cleaning up messes, and after a trip to the bathroom.

For children, the routine is much the same, CDC advises. Center staff should be sure that children's hands are washed when they arrive, before they eat or drink, and after they use the toilet or have their diapers changed.

It's also important that the diaper-changing area is located well away from food-serving areas and that a separate sink is used for preparing food and washing dishes.

CDC recommends that only washable, preferably hard-surfaced toys be used around children still in diapers. Toys should be washed daily. Stuffed toys, if they're used by children in diapers, should be washed at least once a week.

Obviously, the need for cleanliness is not limited to hands and playthings. All facilities and supplies at day-care centers should be washed with soap and water and then disinfected on a regular, frequent schedule. For disinfectants, CDC recommends either a commercial product that kills bacteria, viruses, and parasites such as Giardia or a bleach solution. To make the bleach solution, mix one-fourth cup of bleach with a gallon of water (or one tablespoon per quart). The solution should be made daily but can be stored in a spray bottle. Disinfectants must be kept out of the reach of children.

Any parent knows how disagreeable even a short bout of diarrhea can be in a young child. But public health workers know that diseases spread from day-care centers can have further, more ominous consequences. A day-care center child who contracts hepatitis A, for example, will probably develop only mild symptoms or none at all. Spread to adult family members, however, the infection carries the risk of more serious illness, as well as the possibility of further transmission to the community, particularly if the adult handles or prepares food. According to the National Restaurant Association, there are 8 million food service workers in 550,000 establishments in this country. It is easy to see how enteric disease in a day-care center child can have far-reaching effects into a wider world. In two studies, 13 percent to 40 percent of reported cases of hepatitis A in the community had some form of association with outbreaks in day-care centers.

FDA has model sanitation and food protection codes to which commercial food establishments must adhere. These same codes should apply to day-care centers that handle food, even though centers are not regulated by FDA. At FDA's urging, the National Environmental Health Association devoted its 1987 annual mid-year conference to day-care problems, particularly those associated with food protection and sanitation. The agency also recently signed a memorandum of understanding with the Department of Health and Human Service's Head Start Bureau. It provides for increased cooperation between Head Start and FDA's Center for Food Safety and Applied Nutrition to ensure that day-care centers follow standard sanitation and food protection requirements. And FDA continues to work closely with local and state regulators of day-care centers who are responsible for inspecting these facilities to help ensure that standard public health guidelines are being met.

My advice to parents of day-care center toddlers is: Make sure the day-care center is on guard against contamination that can make your child, you, and lots of other people needlessly sick. The risk is not just a bout of diarrhea. The risk is serious health problems down the road that can—and should—be prevented.

Updated Information on FDA Food Codes

Since the publication of the FDA Consumer article in 1989, FDA has updated model codes related to the preparation of food in food establishments. This update is currently embodied in the 1998 FDA Food Code and is intended to apply to childcare centers. There are several noteworthy provisions in that Code which can help prevent the spread of foodborne diseases:

- Child care center operators must maintain oversight of their employees who prepare food to ensure that those who are ill or exhibit certain symptoms associated with foodborne illness do not prepare food or engage in other activities that could contaminate the food.

- Employees who prepare food are required to report certain symptoms, illnesses, and high-risk conditions related to foodborne illness with which they may have been associated.

- The Code specifies an acceptable method for food employee handwashing during the preparation of food and special hand-washing products (washing twice and using a nailbrush) that are necessary in certain situations, e.g., after using the toilet.

- Touching ready-to-eat food with bare hands is prohibited. Proper utensils or single-service gloves may be used to satisfy this requirement.

- In order to destroy disease-causing organisms, potentially hazardous foods (this means those that can support the growth of disease-causing organisms and includes many foods like cut melons, boiled potatoes, fried rice, and others that you might not think could be dangerous must be:

  1. Cooked to certain temperatures for 15 seconds, depending on the type of food;

  2. Held cold at 41 degrees F or less or hot at 140 degrees F; and

  3. Reheated rapidly to at least 165 degrees F.

- Consult the FDA Food Code for specific temperature requirements and for special provisions related to microwave cooking and reheating.

Young children attending childcare centers are particularly susceptible to foodborne illness and special precautions apply. For example: individual packages of food, like crackers, must not be reserved if they are not eaten, even if they remain unopened; and pasteurized eggs should be used instead of shell eggs.

— by Frank E. Young, M.D., Ph.D,
Commissioner of Food and Drugs

Part Five

The Government's Role in Food Safety

Chapter 48

Progress Report for Food and Drug Safety

On September 26, 1995, the Public Health Service (PHS) conducted a review of progress on HEALTHY PEOPLE 2000 objectives in the Food and Drug Safety priority area.

The Food and Drug Administration (FDA) is the designated PHS lead agency for the Food and Drug Safety priority area. The Deputy Administrator of the U.S. Department of Agriculture's (USDA) Food Safety and Inspection Service (FSIS) participated in the Progress Review. The National Institutes of Health (NIH), Indian Health Service (IHS), Centers for Disease Control and Prevention (CDC), Agency for Health Care Policy and Research (AHCPR), and Health Care Financing Administration (HCFA) were also represented. Guests included the American Medical Association, American Nurses Association, Conference for Food Protection, National Council on Patient Information and Education, and National Association of Boards of Pharmacy.

The progress review focused attention on the importance of FDA's Hazard Analysis Critical Control Point (HACCP) approach to food safety and efforts underway to make this food safety system standard in the U.S. food supply. HACCP employs a science-based analysis of potential hazards, determining where problems can occur and instituting measures to prevent or correct such occurrences.

Objectives 12.1-4 relate to reducing the incidence of foodborne illnesses, encouraging safe food preparation practices, and extending

U.S. Department of Health and Human Services, 1995.

265

the adoption of model food codes. As reported in the April 12, 1995, issue of the *Journal of the American Medical Association*, there was a reduction in the observed incidence of listeriosis between 1989 and 1993, largely as a result of industry, regulatory, and educational efforts conducted by public and private sector organizations working together. Replication of this success for other pathogens may not be possible, owing to the changing epidemiology of foodborne diseases, increased consumer demand for fresh foods year-round, and the appearance of emerging pathogens in new products. In addition, current surveillance systems may not be able to detect changes in incidence. For example, not all States require the reporting of *E. coli* 0157 and *Campylobacter* infections.

A decreasing trend in the number of *Salmonella enteritidis* outbreaks has also been detected and may be associated with the adoption of quality assurance programs by egg producers. Because the elderly and the immunocompromised are more susceptible to salmonellosis, FDA has worked with HCFA to encourage safe food preparation practices and the use of pasteurized eggs in nursing homes.

FDA and USDA/FSIS issued regulatory proposals that would require seafood processing plants and federally inspected meat and poultry plants to adopt HACCP systems for documenting production of safe products. FDA has approved irradiation for use with poultry products. A petition for use of irradiation in other meat products is now under review.

On the basis of a Memorandum of Understanding between FDA and the conference for Food Protection, the Food Code is being reviewed by the conference. FDA plans to revise the Food Code every 2 years. To promote adoption of the Code by States and professional and trade groups, FDA initiated regional training programs in 1994, made presentations before more than 50 audiences that year and, with USDA, conducted four video satellite teleconferences directed at State and local officials. To assist in implementing the Code, the agency has completed development of its Electronic Inspection System (EIS), which provides findings to food establishment operators more efficiently. The IHS representative noted that the incidence of gastrointestinal illnesses had declined by 81 percent since 1974 among American Indians and Alaska Natives, reflecting to a large degree the success of educational efforts directed at foodhandlers.

Participants in the progress review then turned to drug safety issues. It was noted that 98 percent of all pharmacies are now computerized and have the capacity to be linked to centralized databases. Efforts to implement computerized patient records and potential impacts that this technological advance will have on the interaction between health professionals and their patients were discussed.

Objective 12.6 was expanded in the 1995 Midcourse Review to include drug profile reviews by dispensers of medication. In 1992, the Primary Care Providers Survey indicated that 84 percent of internists and 70 percent of family physicians surveyed maintained a current medication list for 81-100 percent of their patients 65 and older. A survey conducted in 1993 by the National Association of Retail Druggists, while not specifically focusing on the age group targeted in objective 12.6, showed that 92 percent of pharmacists queried reported that they provided printed patient drug information. A 1994 study by the National Association of Boards of Pharmacy found that 64 percent of consumers stated that they had received printed material about their medications from the pharmacy. While it was acknowledged that this upward trend in pharmacy-provided information may be due in part to implementation of requirements of the Omnibus Budget Reconciliation Act of 1990, representatives for the profession of pharmacy stressed that this observation is consistent with current shifts in the practice of pharmacy toward a concept of patient advocacy and total care.

In 1993, the FDA MedWatch program was launched to inform health professionals about the importance of monitoring for adverse events and product problems and to facilitate voluntary reporting of such events directly to the agency. The *FDA Desk Guide for Adverse Event and Product Problem Reporting*, which contains reporting forms and instructions for health professionals, can be requested by calling 1-800-FDA-1088. There was an initial mailing of the *Desk Guide* to approximately one-half of all internists in the United States during 1993. The MedWatch reporting form has been published in many widely used drug information sources, such as the *Physicians' Desk Reference*, American Medical Association (AMA) *Drug Evaluations*, and U.S. Pharmacopoeia *Dispensing Information*. For 1994, FDA estimates that 71.6 percent of the adverse drug event reports received by the agency were interpreted as serious. FDA reported that over 100 organizations representing both health professionals and industry have joined as partners to promote the effective use of the MedWatch program.

The discussion focused on the need to ensure the consistent quality and usefulness of printed information being provided to patients concerning the medications they take. It was noted that AHCPR has an initiative in progress designed to acquaint beneficiaries with the types and scope of information they should expect to receive during encounters with physicians and pharmacists. AHCPR noted that we are faced with a significant technical challenge by the increasing need to share information about patients while preserving the patient's right to confidentiality.

The progress review concluded with a call for greater efforts in the areas of both consumer and provider education. There is, as well, a need to strengthen collaboration among Federal agencies (Administration on Aging, for example) and between the Federal sector and professional and patient organizations. Several issues could be brought into sharper focus by research, including how information provided to patients can lead to better health outcomes.

Chapter 49

Foodborne Diseases Active Surveillance Network (FoodNet)

The Foodborne Diseases Active Surveillance Network (FoodNet) is the foodborne disease component of the Emerging Infections Program (EIP) of the Centers for Disease Control and Prevention (CDC). A collaborative project of CDC, the seven EIP sites, the U.S. Department of Agriculture (USDA), and the U.S. Food and Drug Administration (FDA), FoodNet consists of active surveillance for foodborne diseases and related epidemiologic studies designed to help public health officials better understand the epidemiology of foodborne diseases in the United States. FoodNet was established in 1995 in five locations: Minnesota, Oregon, and selected counties in Georgia, California, and Connecticut. The total population of these sites, or catchment areas, is 14.7 million, or 6% of the population of the United States. FoodNet was expanded to selected counties in Maryland and New York in 1997. The goals of FoodNet are to describe the epidemiology of new and reemerging bacterial, parasitic, and viral foodborne pathogens; estimate the frequency and severity of foodborne diseases that occur in the United States per year; and determine how much foodborne illness results from eating specific foods, such as meat, poultry, and eggs.

Foodborne diseases are common; an estimated 6 to 33 million cases occur each year in the United States. Although most of these infections cause mild illness, severe infections and serious complications

Emerging Infectious Diseases Vol 3, No. 4, October-December 1997, National Center for Infectious Diseases, Centers for Disease Control and Prevention, Atlanta, GA.

do occur. The public health challenges of foodborne diseases are changing rapidly; in recent years, new and reemerging foodborne pathogens have been described, and changes in food production have led to new food safety concerns. Foodborne diseases have been associated with many different foods, including some previously thought to be safe, such as eggs and fruit juice, both of which have transmitted Salmonella during recent outbreaks. Public health officials in the seven EIP sites are monitoring foodborne diseases, conducting epidemiologic and laboratory studies of these diseases, and responding to new challenges from these diseases. Information gained through this network will lead to new interventions and prevention strategies for addressing the public health problem of foodborne diseases.

Current "passive" surveillance systems rely upon reporting of foodborne diseases by clinical microbiology laboratories to state health departments, which in turn report to CDC. Although foodborne diseases are extremely common, only a fraction of them are routinely reported to CDC through these surveillance systems. Inadequate reporting results from a complex chain of events that must occur before a case is reported, and a break at any linkage along the chain results in a case not being reported. FoodNet is an "active" surveillance system, meaning public health officials frequently contact microbiology laboratory directors to find new cases of foodborne diseases and report these cases electronically to CDC. In addition, FoodNet is designed to monitor each of the events that occurs along the foodborne diseases pyramid and thereby allow more accurate and precise estimates and interpretation of the prevalence of foodborne diseases over time. Because most foodborne infections cause diarrheal illness, FoodNet focuses these efforts on persons who have a diarrheal illness.

FoodNet Components

Active Laboratory-Based Surveillance

The core of FoodNet is population-based active surveillance at over 300 clinical microbiology laboratories that test stool samples in the seven participating sites. In active surveillance, the laboratories in the catchment areas are contacted regularly by collaborative FoodNet investigators to collect information on all laboratory-confirmed cases of diarrheal illness. Since January 1996, information has been collected on every laboratory-diagnosed case of *Salmonella, Shigella, Campylobacter, Escherichia coli* O157, *Listeria, Yersinia,* and *Vibrio* infection among residents of the catchment areas of the five original sites; this information is transmitted electronically to CDC. The result is a comprehensive and timely database of foodborne illness in a well-defined population.

Survey of Clinical Laboratories

In October 1995, collaborative FoodNet investigators conducted a baseline laboratory survey of all microbiology laboratories in the five original catchment areas to determine which pathogens are included in routine bacterial stool cultures, which tests must be specifically requested by the physician, and what specific techniques are used to isolate the pathogens. A baseline survey will be conducted in the two new sites, and a follow-up survey to assess any recent changes in laboratory practices was conducted in the original sites in 1997. Practices in clinical laboratories have been found to vary; some laboratories look for a wider variety of bacteria than others. The methods used to collect and examine specimens are being investigated because these can influence whether the laboratory finds disease-causing bacteria.

Survey of Physicians

To obtain information on physician stool-culturing practices, collaborative FoodNet investigators mailed a survey questionnaire to 5,000 physicians during 1996. Analysis of these data is ongoing. Because laboratories test stool specimens from a patient only upon the request of a physician or other health-care provider, it is important to measure how often and under what circumstances physicians order these tests. As changes occur in the way health care is provided in the United States, stool-culturing practices may also change. The practices of physicians who send stool samples to laboratories within the catchment areas will be monitored by surveys and validation studies.

Survey of the Population

Collaborative FoodNet investigators contact randomly selected residents of a catchment area and ask whether the person has had a recent diarrheal illness, whether the person sought treatment for the illness, and whether the person had consumed certain foods known to have caused outbreaks of foodborne illness. During 1996, 750 residents of the catchment areas were interviewed by telephone each month (9,000/year). Because many who become ill with diarrhea do not see a physician, little is known about the number of cases of diarrhea in the general population and how often persons with diarrhea

271

seek medical care. The population survey is an essential part of active surveillance for foodborne illness because it allows for an estimate of the population who seeks medical care when affected by diarrheal illness.

Case-Control Studies

In 1996, the FoodNet began case-control studies of *E. coli* O157 and *Salmonella* serogroup B and D infections. More than 60% of *Salmonella* infections in the United States are caused by serogroup B and D *Salmonella*. These large case-control studies will provide new and more precise information about which food items or other exposures may cause these diseases. To allow the most precise classification of the isolates from the patients in these studies, the Salmonella and *E. coli* O157:H7 laboratory specimens from these patients are sent from FoodNet sites to CDC for further study, including antibiotic resistance testing, phage typing, and molecular subtyping.

Accomplishments

Since becoming operational on January 1, 1996, FoodNet has tracked the rates of foodborne diseases. Even in the first year of data collection, numerous interesting patterns and outbreaks were detected. Surprisingly high isolation rates for *Y. enterocolitica* in Georgia and *Campylobacter* in California were detected. An outbreak of *Salmonella* infections caused by contaminated alfalfa sprouts was detected in Oregon. Two outbreaks of *E. coli* O157:H7 infections were detected in Connecticut, one due to lettuce and one to apple cider. FoodNet has also provided the infrastructure for conducting active surveillance for new and reemerging diseases. When an association between bovine spongiform encephalopathy in cattle and variant_Creutzfeldt-Jakob disease in humans was suspected in the United Kingdom, EIP personnel conducted surveillance for this rare human disease. EIP personnel also collaborated in the investigation of a multistate outbreak of *Cyclospora* infections associated with consumption of raspberries from Guatemala.

Chapter 50

National Computer Network in Place to Combat Foodborne Illness (PulseNet)

HHS Secretary Donna E. Shalala announced completion of PulseNet, a national computer network of public health laboratories that will help rapidly identify and stop episodes of foodborne illness. The new system enables epidemiologists to move up to five times faster than previously feasible in identifying serious and wide-spread food contamination problems.

Speaking at a White House event with Vice President Al Gore, Secretary Shalala said the new national PulseNet system is the latest feature of the Clinton administration's initiative to improve food safety and detect foodborne disease. She said the next step should be increased resources for food safety efforts, and legislation to help ensure the safety of imported foods.

"America's food supply is unmatched in quality and quantity, but we face new challenges as our food distribution systems change and as new pathogens emerge and familiar ones grow resistant to treatment," Shalala said. "PulseNet will help us keep ahead of these challenges. We also need action by Congress to increase food safety resources at CDC and the Food and Drug Administration, and to pass legislation that will give FDA authority to ensure the safety of imported foods."

PulseNet is based on a molecular technology called pulsed-field gel electrophoresis (PFGE), standardized by HHS' Centers for Disease Control and Prevention, to identify distinctive "fingerprint" patterns

HHS News, May 1998; U.S. Department of Health and Human Services.

of *E. coli* O157:H7. Under the networked computer system officially launched today, public health laboratories throughout the country can use this technology and share information via the Internet to determine when foodborne disease outbreaks are occurring. In this way, epidemiologists are able to rapidly assess whether a widespread food incident is underway, and can more quickly trace the source of the problem.

"Foods reaching American tables today are produced, processed and distributed very differently from even a decade ago. Food from a single source may be rapidly distributed to communities across the nation, making it more difficult to detect a disease outbreak caused by a contaminated food product," Secretary Shalala said. "PulseNet combines the latest in microbiology and computer technology to quickly detect whether illness occurring in many different locations, during the same timeframe, are linked to a common food source."

The PFGE technology underlying PulseNet was first used by CDC in a foodborne illness outbreak in 1993, but lack of computer networking prevented the rapid response that is possible today. Computer networking began with public health labs in four states in 1995, and has recently been expanded to 12 additional states.

This announcement marks the ability of the four key area laboratories, as well as U.S. Department of Agriculture and Food And Drug Administration labs, to link directly with the CDC computer server and gain direct access to the CDC database, allowing rapid direct exchange of information.

"With these computer links, the PulseNet system is in place, and its full technical potential is available to help protect Americans from foodborne illness," Secretary Shalala said.

The PulseNet computer network grew out of the experience of public health experts when investigating a large outbreak of foodborne illness caused by a deadly strain of bacteria, *E.coli* O157:H7, in 1993. Today, what takes as little as 48 hours with PulseNet took weeks in 1993 as investigators searched for the common food source of the outbreak—ultimately determined to be hamburger patties served at a large chain of regional fast food restaurants.

In the 1993 outbreak, CDC scientists performed the relatively new technique of DNA "fingerprinting" and determined the strain of *E. coli* O157:H7 found in patients matched the strain found in hamburger patties—the source of the outbreak. The prompt recall of the suspected ground beef patties prevented an estimated 800 additional illnesses in 1993; however, more than 700 persons became ill and 4 children died in the outbreak. The process of matching the bacterial strains in multiple communities was slowed because public health labs in multiple states could not quickly share information about their samples of *E. coli*. Now, with PulseNet, labs can instantly determine if a sample of the *E. coli* strain causing illness in their communities is also causing illness in communities next door or across the country.

"PulseNet can help public health experts recognize that foodborne illness occurring at the same time but in widely dispersed locations are from the same strain, and may be from a common exposure," said acting CDC Director Claire Broome, M.D. "By matching bacteria subtype patterns, we can detect nationwide outbreaks quickly and better direct public health actions."

Because bacteria replicate themselves by dividing in two, the next generation and many after have the same or nearly the same genetic makeup as the parent bacterium. The similarity of genetic materials over generations makes this an excellent tool to identify outbreaks from a common source, including food. Today PulseNet participants perform DNA fingerprinting on *E. coli* O157:H7 isolates. In the near future, another bacterium that is an important cause of foodborne illness, *Salmonella* serotype Typhimurium, will be added to PulseNet. Over time, CDC will set up additional databases of DNA fingerprints for other bacteria that can cause illness through food.

Federal food safety agencies worked with the Association of State and Territorial Public Health Laboratory Directors in creating PulseNet. In 1995, CDC began to set up PulseNet with state public health laboratories in Massachusetts, Minnesota, Texas and Washington, which are designated area laboratories and provide PulseNet services to states in their region. In addition, USDA and FDA have come on-line.

Additional laboratories are joining CDC's PulseNet. In addition to the four area laboratories directly linked to CDC, other labs connected to PulseNet include those from California, Colorado, Florida, Georgia, Iowa, New Hampshire, New York, Ohio, Oregon, Utah, Virginia and Wisconsin.

Part Six

Additional Help and Resources

Chapter 51

Glossary

A

Abdomen: The area between the chest and the hips. Contains the stomach, small intestine, large intestine, liver, gallbladder, pancreas, and spleen.

Absorption: The way nutrients from food move from the small intestine into the cells in the body.

Activated Charcoal: An over-the-counter product that may help relieve intestinal gas.

Acute: A disorder that is sudden and severe but lasts only a short time.

Allergy: A condition in which the body is not able to tolerate certain foods, animals, plants, or other substances.

Amebiasis: An acute or chronic infection. Symptoms vary from mild diarrhea to frequent watery diarrhea and loss of water and fluids in the body. See also Gastroenteritis.

Excerpted from "The Digestive Diseases Dictionary," National Institute of Diabetes and Digestive and Kidney Diseases (NIDDK), NIH Pub. No. 97-2750, March 1997.

279

Antacids: Medicines that balance acids and gas in the stomach. Examples are Maalox, Mylanta, and Di-Gel.

Anticholinergics: Medicines that calm muscle spasms in the intestine. Examples are dicyclomine (dy-SY-kloh-meen) (Bentyl) and hyoscyamine (HY-oh-SY-uh-meen) (Levsin).

Antidiarrheals: Medicines that help control diarrhea. An example is loperamide (lo-PEH-ruh-myd) (Imodium).

Antiemetics: Medicines that prevent and control nausea and vomiting. Examples are promethazine (pro-MEH-thuh-zeen) (Phenergan) and prochlorperazine (pro-klor-PEH-ruh-zeen) (Compazine).

Antispasmodics: Medicines that help reduce or stop muscle spasms in the intestines. Examples are dicyclomine (dy-SY-klo-meen) (Bentyl) and atropine (AH-tro-peen) (Donnatal).

Asymptomatic: The condition of having a disease, but without any symptoms of it.

Atrophic Gastritis: Chronic irritation of the stomach lining. Causes the stomach lining and glands to wither away.

B

Bismuth Subsalicylate: A nonprescription medicine such as Pepto-Bismol. Used to treat diarrhea, heartburn, indigestion, and nausea. It is also part of the treatment for ulcers caused by the bacterium *Helicobacter pylori*.

Bloating: Fullness or swelling in the abdomen that often occurs after meals.

Borborygmi: Rumbling sounds caused by gas moving through the intestines (stomach "growling").

Bowel: Another word for the small and large intestines.

Bowel Movement: Body wastes passed through the rectum and anus.

Bulking Agents: Laxatives that make bowel movements soft and easy to pass.

C

***Campylobacter pylori*:** The original name for the bacterium that causes ulcers. The new name is *Helicobacter pylori*. See also *Helicobacter pylori*.

Candidiasis: A mild infection caused by the Candida fungus, which lives naturally in the gastrointestinal tract. Infection occurs when a change in the body, such as surgery, causes the fungus to overgrow suddenly.

Cholesterol: A fat-like substance in the body. The body makes and needs some cholesterol, which also comes from foods such as butter and egg yolks. Too much cholesterol may cause gallstones. It also may cause fat to build up in the arteries. This may cause a disease that slows or stops blood flow.

Chronic: A term that refers to disorders that last a long time, often years.

***Clostridium difficile* (*C. difficile*):** Bacteria naturally present in the large intestine. These bacteria make a substance that can cause a serious infection called pseudomembranous colitis in people taking antibiotics.

Colic: Attacks of abdominal pain, caused by muscle spasms in the intestines. Colic is common in infants.

Colitis: Irritation of the colon.

Constipation: A condition in which the stool becomes hard and dry. A person who is constipated usually has fewer than three bowel movements in a week. Bowel movements may be painful.
Common causes of constipation:

- Not enough fiber in diet.
- Not enough liquids.
- Lack of exercise.

- Changes in life or routine such as pregnancy, older age, and travel.
- Ignoring the urge to have a bowel movement.
- Problems with the colon and rectum.
- Problems with intestinal function.
- Irritable bowl syndrome.
- Medications.

Cryptosporidia: A parasite that can cause gastrointestinal infection and diarrhea. See also Gastroenteritis.

Cyclic Vomiting Syndrome (CVS): Sudden, repeated attacks of severe vomiting (especially in children), nausea, and physical exhaustion with no apparent cause. Can last from a few hours to 10 days. The episodes begin and end suddenly. Loss of fluids in the body and changes in chemicals in the body can require immediate medical attention. Also called abdominal migraine.

D

Defecation: The passage of bowel contents through the rectum and anus.

Dehydration: Loss of fluids from the body, often caused by diarrhea. May result in loss of important salts and minerals.

Diarrhea: Frequent, loose, and watery bowel movements. Common causes include gastrointestinal infections, irritable bowel syndrome, medicines, and malabsorption.

Digestants: Medicines that aid or stimulate digestion. An example is a digestive enzyme such as Lactaid for people with lactase deficiency.

Digestion: The process the body uses to break down food into simple substances for energy, growth, and cell repair.

Digestive System: The organs in the body that break down and absorb food. Organs that make up the digestive system are the mouth, esophagus, stomach, small intestine, large intestine, rectum, and anus. Organs that help with digestion but are not part of the digestive tract are the tongue, glands in the mouth that make saliva, pancreas, liver, and gallbladder.

Distention: Bloating or swelling of the abdomen.

Duodenitis: An irritation of the first part of the small intestine (duodenum).

Dysentery: An infectious disease of the colon. Symptoms include bloody, mucus-filled diarrhea; abdominal pain; fever; and loss of fluids from the body.

Dysphagia: Problems in swallowing food or liquid, usually caused by blockage or injury to the esophagus.

E

Encopresis: Accidental passage of a bowel movement. A common disorder in children.

Endoscopy: A procedure that uses an endoscope to diagnose or treat a condition.

Enema: A liquid put into the rectum to clear out the bowel or to administer drugs or food.

Enteritis: An irritation of the small intestine.

Eosinophilic Gastroenteritis: Infection and swelling of the lining of the stomach, small intestine, or large intestine. The infection is caused by white blood cells (eosinophils).

Escherichia coli: Bacteria that cause infection and irritation of the large intestine. The bacteria are spread by unclean water, dirty cooking utensils, or undercooked meat. See also Gastroenteritis.

Esophageal Spasms: Muscle cramps in the esophagus that cause pain in the chest.

F

Fecal Occult Blood Test (FOBT): A test to see whether there is blood in the stool that is not visible to the naked eye. A sample of stool is placed on a chemical strip that will change color if blood is present. Hidden blood in the stool is a common symptom of colorectal cancer.

Fermentation: The process of bacteria breaking down undigested food and releasing alcohols, acids, and gases.

Fiber: A substance in foods that comes from plants. Fiber helps with digestion by keeping stool soft so that it moves smoothly through the colon. Soluble fiber dissolves in water. Soluble fiber is found in beans, fruit, and oat products. Insoluble fiber does not dissolve in water. Insoluble fiber is found in whole-grain products and vegetables.

Flatulence: Excessive gas in the stomach or intestine. May cause bloating.

Foodborne Illness: An acute gastrointestinal infection caused by food that contains harmful bacteria. Symptoms include diarrhea, abdominal pain, fever, and chills. Also called food poisoning.

G

Gas: Air that comes from normal breakdown of food. The gases are passed out of the body through the rectum (flatus) or the mouth (burp).

Gastric: Related to the stomach.

Gastric Juices: Liquids produced in the stomach to help break down food and kill bacteria.

Gastritis: An inflammation of the stomach lining.

Gastroenteritis: An infection or irritation of the stomach and intestines. May be caused by bacteria or parasites from spoiled food or unclean water. Other causes include eating food that irritates the stomach lining and emotional upsets such as anger, fear, or stress. Symptoms include diarrhea, nausea, vomiting, and abdominal cramping. See also Infectious Diarrhea and Travelers' Diarrhea.

Causes of gastroenteritis:

- Bacteria
  - *Escherichia coli.*
  - *Salmonella.*
  - *Shigella.*

- Viruses
  - Norwalk virus.
  - Rotavirus.

- Parasites
  - *Cryptosporidia.*
  - *Entamoeba histolytica.*
  - *Giardia lamblia.*

Gastroenterologist: A doctor who specializes in digestive diseases.

Gastrointestinal (GI) Tract: The large, muscular tube that extends from the mouth to the anus, where the movement of muscles and release of hormones and enzymes digest food. Also called the alimentary canal or digestive tract.

Giardiasis: An infection with the parasite *Giardia lamblia* from spoiled food or unclean water. May cause diarrhea. See also Gastroenteritis.

H

Heartburn: A painful, burning feeling in the chest. Heartburn is caused by stomach acid flowing back into the esophagus. Changing the diet and other habits can help to prevent heartburn. Heartburn may be a symptom of GERD.

> *Tips to control heartburn:* Avoid foods and beverages that affect lower esophageal sphincter pressure or irritate the esophagus lining. Lose weight if overweight. Stop smoking. Elevate the head of the bed 6 inches. Avoid lying down 2 to 3 hours after eating. Take an antacid.

Helicobacter pylori (H. pylori): A spiral-shaped bacterium found in the stomach. *H. pylori* damages stomach and duodenal tissue, causing ulcers. Previously called *Campylobacter pylori.*

Hepatic: Related to the liver.

Hepatitis: Irritation of the liver that sometimes causes permanent damage. Hepatitis may be caused by viruses or by medicines or alcohol. Hepatitis has the following forms:

Hepatitis A: A virus most often spread by unclean food and water.

Hepatitis B: A virus commonly spread by sexual intercourse or blood transfusion, or from mother to newborn at birth. Another way it spreads is by using a needle that was used by an infected person. Hepatitis B is more common and much more easily spread than the AIDS virus and may lead to cirrhosis and liver cancer.

Hepatitis C: A virus spread by blood transfusion and possibly by sexual intercourse or sharing needles with infected people. Hepatitis C may lead to cirrhosis and liver cancer. Hepatitis C used to be called non-A, non-B hepatitis.

Hepatitis D (Delta): A virus that occurs mostly in people who take illegal drugs by using needles. Only people who have hepatitis B can get hepatitis D.

Hepatitis E: A virus spread mostly through unclean water. This type of hepatitis is common in developing countries. It has not occurred in the United States.

Hepatitis B Immunoglobulin (HBIg): A shot that gives short-term protection from the hepatitis B virus.

Hepatitis B Vaccine: A shot to prevent hepatitis B. The vaccine tells the body to make its own protection (antibodies) against the virus.

Hepatotoxicity: How much damage a medicine or other substance does to the liver.

Hydrogen Breath Test: A test for lactose intolerance. It measures breath samples for too much hydrogen. The body makes too much hydrogen when lactose is not broken down properly in the small intestine.

I

lleocolitis: Irritation of the lower part of the small intestine (ileum) and colon.

Indigestion: Poor digestion. Symptoms include heartburn, nausea, bloating, and gas. Also called dyspepsia.

Infectious Diarrhea: Diarrhea caused by infection from bacteria, viruses, or parasites. See also Travelers' Diarrhea and Gastroenteritis.

Infectious Gastroenteritis: See Gastroenteritis.

Intestinal Flora: The bacteria, yeasts, and fungi that grow normally in the intestines.

Intestinal Mucosa: The surface lining of the intestines where the cells absorb nutrients.

J

Jaundice: A symptom of many disorders. Jaundice causes the skin and eyes to turn yellow from too much bilirubin in the blood.

K

Kupffer's Cells: Cells that line the liver. These cells remove waste such as bacteria from the blood.

L

Large Intestine: The part of the intestine that goes from the cecum to the rectum. The large intestine absorbs water from stool and changes it from a liquid to a solid form. The large intestine is 5 feet long and includes the appendix, cecum, colon, and rectum. Also called colon.

Lavage: A cleaning of the stomach and colon. Uses a special drink and enemas.

Laxatives: Medicines to relieve long-term constipation. Used only if other methods fail. Also called cathartics.

Liver: The largest organ in the body. The liver carries out many important functions, such as making bile, changing food into energy, and cleaning alcohol and poisons from the blood.

Liver Enzyme Tests: Blood tests that look at how well the liver and biliary system are working. Also called liver function tests.

Lower GI Series: X-rays of the rectum, colon, and lower part of the small intestine. A barium enema is given first. Barium coats the organs so they will show up on the x-ray. Also called barium enema x-ray.

M

Malabsorption Syndromes: Conditions that happen when the small intestine cannot absorb nutrients from foods.

Metabolism: The way cells change food into energy after food is digested and absorbed into the blood.

Motility: The movement of food through the digestive tract.

Mucosal Protective Drugs: Medicines that protect the stomach lining from acid. Examples are sucralfate (soo-CRAL-fayt) (Carafate), misoprostol (MIH-soh-PROH-stawl) (Cytotec), antacids (Mylanta and Maalox), and bismuth subsalicylate (Pepto-Bismol).

Mucosal Lining: The lining of GI tract organs that makes mucus.

N

Nausea: The feeling of wanting to throw up (vomit).

Norwalk Virus: A virus that may cause GI infection and diarrhea. See also Gastroenteritis.

O

Occult Bleeding: Blood in stool that is not visible to the naked eye. May be a sign of disease such as diverticulosis or colorectal cancer.

P

Pepsin: An enzyme made in the stomach that breaks down proteins.

Peptic: Related to the stomach and the duodenum, where pepsin is present.

Peristalsis: A wavelike movement of muscles in the GI tract. Peristalsis moves food and liquid through the GI tract.

Prokinetic Drugs: Medicines that cause muscles in the GI tract to move food. An example is cisapride (SIS-uh-pryd) (Propulsid).

Protein: One of the three main classes of food. Protein is found in meat, eggs, and beans. The stomach and small intestine break down proteins into amino acids. The blood absorbs amino acids and uses them to build and mend cells.

Pseudomembranous Colitis: Severe irritation of the colon. Caused by *Clostridium difficile* bacteria. Occurs after taking oral antibiotics, which kill bacteria that normally live in the colon.

Pyloric Sphincter: The muscle between the stomach and the small intestine.

Pyloric Stenosis: A narrowing of the opening between the stomach and the small intestine.

Pylorus: The opening from the stomach into the top of the small intestine (duodenum).

R

Rectum: The lower end of the large intestine, leading to the anus.

Reflux: A condition that occurs when gastric juices or small amounts of food from the stomach flow back into the esophagus and mouth. Also called regurgitation.

Reflux Esophagitis: Irritation of the esophagus because stomach contents flow back into the esophagus.

Rotavirus: The most common cause of infectious diarrhea in the United States, especially in children under age 2.

S

Salmonella: A bacterium that may cause intestinal infection and diarrhea. See also Gastroenteritis.

Shigellosis: Infection with the bacterium *Shigella*. Usually causes a high fever, acute diarrhea, and dehydration. See also Gastroenteritis.

Sigmoid Colon: The lower part of the colon that empties into the rectum.

Sigmoidoscopy: Looking into the sigmoid colon and rectum with a flexible or rigid tube, called a sigmoidoscope.

Small Intestine: Organ where most digestion occurs. It measures about 20 feet and includes the duodenum, jejunum, and ileum.

Spasms: Muscle movements such as those in the colon that cause pain, cramps, and diarrhea.

Spleen: The organ that cleans blood and makes white blood cells. White blood cells attack bacteria and other foreign cells.

Stomach: The organ between the esophagus and the small intestine. The stomach is where digestion of protein begins.

Stool: The solid wastes that pass through the rectum as bowel movements. Stools are undigested foods, bacteria, mucus, and dead cells. Also called feces.

T

Transverse Colon: The part of the colon that goes across the abdomen from right to left.

Traveler's Diarrhea: An infection caused by unclean food or drink. Often occurs during travel outside one's own country. See also Gastroenteritis.

Triple-Therapy: A combination of three medicines used to treat *Helicobacter pylori* infection and ulcers. Drugs that stop the body from making acid are often added to relieve symptoms.

U

Upper GI Series: X-rays of the esophagus, stomach, and duodenum. The patient swallows barium first. Barium makes the organs show up on x-rays. Also called barium meal.

Urea Breath Test: A test used to detect *Helicobacter pylori* infection. The test measures breath samples for urease, an enzyme *H. pylori* makes.

V

Viral Hepatitis: Hepatitis caused by a virus. Five different viruses (A, B, C, D, and E) most commonly cause this form of hepatitis. Other rare viruses may also cause hepatitis. See Hepatitis.

Type of Hepatitis	Mode of Transmission
Hepatitis A	Contaminated food and water.
Hepatitis B	Sexual intercourse; Sharing infected needles.
Hepatitis C	Sexual intercourse; Sharing infected needles.
Hepatitis D	Must have hepatitis B; Found mainly in intravenous drug users.
Hepatitis E	Contaminated water from poor sanitation.

Vomiting: The release of stomach contents through the mouth.

Chapter 52

Food Safety:
A Team Approach

The United States maintains one of the world's safest food supplies, thanks in large part to an interlocking monitoring system that watches over food production and distribution at every level-locally, statewide and nationally.

Continual monitoring is provided by food inspectors, microbiologists, epidemiologists, and other food scientists working for city and county health departments, state public health agencies, and various federal departments and agencies. Their precise duties are dictated by local, state and national laws, guidelines and other directives. Some monitor only one kind of food, such as milk or seafood. Others work strictly within a specified geographic area. Others are responsible for only one type of food establishment, such as restaurants or meatpacking plants. Together they make up the U.S. food safety team.

The Clinton administration's Food Safety Initiative, begun in 1997, strengthens the efforts of all the members of the nation's food safety team in the fight against food-borne illness, which afflicts between 6.5 million and 33 million Americans every year. One of the initiative's major programs got under way in May 1998 when the Department of Health and Human Services (which includes FDA), the U.S. Department of Agriculture, and the Environmental Protection Agency signed a memorandum of understanding to create a Food Outbreak Response Coordinating Group, or FORC-G. The new group will:

Food and Drug Administration, September 24, 1998.

293

- increase coordination and communication among federal, state and local food

- safety agencies

- guide efficient use of resources and expertise during an outbreak

- prepare for new and emerging threats to the U.S. food supply.

Besides federal officials, members of FORC-G include the Association of Food and Drug Officials, National Association of City and County Health Officials, Association of State and Territorial Public Health Laboratory Directors, Council of State and Territorial Epidemiologists, and National Association of State Departments of Agriculture.

The following table offers a closer look at the nation's food safety lineup. The agencies listed in the table also work with other government agencies, such as the Consumer Product Safety Commission to enforce the Poison Prevention Packaging Act, the FBI to enforce the Federal Anti-Tampering Act, the Department of Transportation to enforce the Sanitary Food Transportation Act, and the U.S. Postal Service to enforce laws against mail fraud.

U.S. Department of Health and Human Services

Food and Drug Administration

Oversees

- All domestic and imported food sold in interstate commerce, including shell eggs, but not meat and poultry

- Bottled water

- Wine beverages with less than 7 percent alcohol

Food Safety Role

Enforces food safety laws governing domestic and imported food, except meat and poultry, by:

- Inspecting food production establishments and food warehouses and collecting and analyzing samples for physical, chemical and microbial contamination

- Reviewing safety of food and color additives before marketing

- Reviewing animal drugs for safety to animals that receive them and humans who eat food produced from the animals

- Monitoring safety of animal feeds used in food-producing animals

- Developing model codes and ordinances, guidelines and interpretations and working with states to implement them in regulating milk and shellfish and retail food establishments, such as restaurants and grocery stores. An example is the model Food Code, a reference for retail outlets and nursing homes and other institutions on how to prepare food to prevent food-borne illness.

- Establishing good food manufacturing practices and other production standards, such as plant sanitation, packaging requirements, and Hazard Analysis and Critical Control Point programs

- Working with foreign governments to ensure safety of certain imported food products

- Requesting manufacturers to recall unsafe food products and monitoring those recalls

- Taking appropriate enforcement actions

- Conducting research on food safety

- Educating industry and consumers on safe food handling practices

For More Information

Consumers:
FDA Headquarters
Office of Consumer Affairs
HFE-88
5600 Fishers Lane
Rockville, MD 20857

Regional FDA offices, listed in the blue pages of the phone book under U.S. Government

Media inquiries: 202-205-4144

Consumers:
FDA's Food Information and Seafood Hotline
1-800-FDA-4010 (1-800-332-4010),
202-205-4314 in the Washington, D.C., area
www.cfsan.fda.gov/list.html
www.fda.gov/cvm/

Centers for Disease Control and Prevention

Oversees

- All foods

Food Safety Role

- Investigates with local, state and other federal officials sources of food-borne disease outbreaks

- Maintains a nationwide system of food-borne disease surveillance: Designs and puts in place rapid, electronic systems for reporting food-borne infections. Works with other federal and state agencies to monitor rates of and trends in food-borne disease outbreaks. Develops state-of-the-art techniques for rapid identification of food-borne pathogens at the state and local levels.

- Develops and advocates public health policies to prevent food-borne diseases

- Conducts research to help prevent food-borne illness

- Trains local and state food safety personnel

For More Information

Centers for Disease Control and Prevention
1600 Clifton Rd., N.E.
Atlanta, GA 30333

Media inquiries: 404-639-3286

General public: 404-639-3311

Website: www.cdc.gov

U.S. Department of Agriculture

Food Safety and Inspection Service

Oversees

- Domestic and imported meat and poultry and related products, such as meat- or poultry-containing stews, pizzas and frozen foods

- Processed egg products (generally liquid, frozen and dried pasteurized egg products)

Food Safety Role

Enforces food safety laws governing domestic and imported meat and poultry products by:

- Inspecting food animals for diseases before and after slaughter

- Inspecting meat and poultry slaughter and processing plants

- With USDA's Agricultural Marketing Service, monitoring and inspecting processed egg products

- Collecting and analyzing samples of food products for microbial and chemical contaminants and infectious and toxic agents

- Establishing production standards for use of food additives and other ingredients in preparing and packaging meat and poultry products, plant sanitation, thermal processing, and other processes

- Making sure all foreign meat and poultry processing plants exporting to the United States meet U.S. standards

- Seeking voluntary recalls by meat and poultry processors of unsafe products

- Sponsoring research on meat and poultry safety

- Educating industry and consumers on safe food-handling practices

For More Information

FSIS Food Safety Education and Communications Staff
Room 1175, South Building,
1400 Independence Ave., S.W.
Washington, DC 20250

Media inquiries: 202-720-9113

Consumers:
The Meat and Poultry Hotline, 1-800-535-4555
(In Washington, D.C., area, call 202-720-3333)
TDD/TTY: 1-800-256-7072
www.fsis.usda.gov

Cooperative State Research, Education, and Extension Service

Oversees

- All domestic foods, some imported

Food Safety Role

- With U.S. colleges and universities, develops research and education programs on food safety for farmers and consumers

For More Information

Local cooperative extension services, listed in the blue pages of the phone book under county government

Cooperative State Research, Education and Extension Service
U.S. Department of Agriculture
Washington, DC 20250-0900; 202-720-3029
www.reeusda.gov

National Agricultural Library

USDA/FDA Foodborne Illness Education Information Center

Oversees

- All foods

Food Safety Role

- Maintains a database of computer software, audiovisuals, posters, games, teachers' guides and other educational materials on preventing food-borne illness
- Helps educators, food service trainers and consumers locate educational materials on preventing food-borne illness

For More Information

USDA/FDA Foodborne Illness Education Information Center
Food and Nutrition Information Center
National Agricultural Library/USDA
Beltsville, MD 20705-2351; 301-504-5719
www.nal.usda.gov/fnic/

U.S. Environmental Protection Agency

Oversees

- Drinking water

Food Safety Role

- Foods made from plants, seafood, meat and poultry
- Establishes safe drinking water standards
- Regulates toxic substances and wastes to prevent their entry into the environment and food chain
- Assists states in monitoring quality of drinking water and finding ways to prevent contamination of drinking water
- Determines safety of new pesticides, sets tolerance levels for pesticide residues in foods, and publishes directions on safe use of pesticides

For More Information

Environmental Protection Agency
401 M St., S.W.
Washington, DC 20460
202-260-2090

Regional EPA offices, listed in the blue pages of the phone book under U.S. Government

www.epa.gov

U.S. Department of Commerce

National Oceanic and Atmospheric Administration

Oversees

- Fish and seafood products

Food Safety Role

- Through its fee-for-service Seafood Inspection Program, inspects and certifies fishing vessels, seafood processing plants, and retail facilities for federal sanitation standards

For More Information

Seafood Inspection Program
1315 East-West Highway
Silver Spring, MD 20910
1-800-422-2750
www.nmfs.gov/iss/services.html

U.S. Department of the Treasury

Bureau of Alcohol, Tobacco and Firearms

Oversees

- Alcoholic beverages except wine beverages containing less than 7 percent alcohol

Food Safety Role

- Enforces food safety laws governing production and distribution of alcoholic beverages

- Investigates cases of adulterated alcoholic products, sometimes with help from FDA

For More Information

Bureau of Alcohol, Tobacco and Firearms
Market Compliance Branch
650 Massachusetts Ave., N.W., Room 5200
Washington, DC 20226
202-927-8130
www.atf.treas.gov/core/alcohol/alcohol.htm

U.S. Customs Service

Oversees

- Imported foods

Food Safety Role

- Works with federal regulatory agencies to ensure that all goods entering and exiting the United States do so according to U.S. laws and regulations

For More Information

U.S. Customs Service
P.O. Box 7407
Washington, DC 20044

Media inquiries: 202-927-1770

General public: Contact local ports of entry, listed in the blue pages of the phone book under U.S. Government, Customs Services

www.customs.ustreas.gov

U.S. Department of Justice

Oversees

• All foods

Food Safety Role

• Prosecutes companies and individuals suspected of violating food safety laws Through U.S. Marshals Service, seizes unsafe food products not yet in the marketplace, as ordered by courts

For More Information

U.S. attorneys' offices in blue pages of phone book under U.S. Government

www.usdoj.gov

Federal Trade Commission

Oversees

• All foods

Food Safety Role

• Enforces a variety of laws that protect consumers from unfair, deceptive or fraudulent practices, including deceptive and unsubstantiated advertising.

For More Information

FTC (Federal Trade Commission)
Consumer Response Center, CRC-240
Washington, DC 20580

Media inquiries: 202-326-2180
TDD: 202-326-2502

Consumers: 202-FTC-HELP
(202-382-4357)

www.ftc.gov

State and Local Governments

Oversees

- All foods within their jurisdictions

Food Safety Role

- Work with FDA and other federal agencies to implement food safety standards for fish, seafood, milk, and other foods produced within state borders
- Inspect restaurants, grocery stores, and other retail food establishments, as well as dairy farms and milk processing plants, grain mills, and food manufacturing plants within local jurisdictions
- Embargo (stop the sale of) unsafe food products made or distributed within state borders

For More Information

City, county and state health, agriculture and environmental protection agencies, listed in the blue pages of the phone book under city, county and state government

Chapter 53

What to Do If You Have a Problem with Food Products

Problems:

- Your hot dog has a strip of plastic inside.
- The canned chili contains a metal washer.
- You think a restaurant dinner made you ill.
- A sugar-coated roach was in your box of cereal.

What can you do?

For Help with Meat, Poultry and Egg Products

Call the toll-free USDA Meat and Poultry Hotline at:
1 (800) 535-4555

For Help with Restaurant Food Problems:

Call the Health Department in your city, county or state.

For Help with Non-Meat Food Products:

For complaints about food products which do not contain meat or poultry—such as cereal—call or write to the Food and Drug Administration

---

Consumer Education and Information, May 1996; Food Safety and Inspection Service, United States Department of Agriculture, Washington, D.C. 20250-3700.

(FDA). Check your local phone book under U.S. Government, Health and Human Services, to find an FDA office in your area.

The FDA's Seafood Hotline is at 1 (800) 332-4010.

In Order for the USDA to Investigate a Problem with Meat, Poultry or Egg Products, You Must Have:

- the original container or packaging;

- the foreign object (the plastic strip or metal washer, for example); and any uneaten portion of the food (refrigerate or freeze it).

Information You Should Be Ready to Tell the Hotline On the Phone Includes:

- your name, address and phone number;

- the brand name, product name and manufacturer of the product;

- the size and package type;

- can or package codes (not UPC bar codes) and dates;

- establishment number (EST) usually found in the circle or shield near the "USDA passed and inspected" phrase;

- name and location of store and date you purchased the product.

You can complain to the store or the product's manufacturer if you don't choose to make a formal complaint to the USDA.

If You Think You Are Ill, See a Physician.

- If an injury or illness allegedly resulted from use of a meat or poultry product, you will also need to tell the Hotline staff about the type, symptoms, time of occurrence and name of attending health professional (if applicable).

- If you can't reach the Hotline staff, or if an injury or illness allegedly resulted from restaurant food, call your local the Health Department.

- If an injury or illness allegedly resulted from non-meat food products, call or write to the FDA.

The Bottom Line:

If you sense there's a problem with any food product, don't consume it. "When in doubt, throw it out."

For Further Information Contact:

FSIS Food Safety Education and Communications Staff
Meat and Poultry Hotline:
1-800-535-4555 (Tollfree Nationwide)
(202) 720-3333 (Washington, DC area)
1-800-256-7072 (TDD/TTY)

Chapter 54

Obtaining the 1999 Food Code

Introduction

The Food and Drug Administration publishes the Food Code, a reference that guides retail outlets such as restaurants and grocery stores and institutions such as nursing homes on how to prevent foodborne illness.

Local, state and federal regulators use the FDA Food Code as a model to help develop or update their own food safety rules and to be consistent with national food regulatory policy. Also, many of the over 1 million retail food establishments apply Food Code provisions to their own operations.

The Food Code is updated every two years, to coincide with the biennial meeting of the Conference for Food Protection. The conference is a group of representatives from regulatory agencies at all levels of government, the food industry, academia, and consumer organizations that works to improve food safety at the retail level.

Obtaining the 1999 Food Code

Copies of the 1999 Food Code are available in the following formats. Downloaded documents can be accessed through FDA's website at www.fda.gov:

U. S. Department of Health and Human Services; Public Health Service; Food and Drug Administration.

- 1999 Food Code in HTML or PDF versions.

  Summary of Changes

- Download the full 1999 Food Code in PDF format. (1Mb; 1.2Mb uncompressed)

  (Obtain a PDF reader.)

- Word Perfect 6/7/8 version compressed in self-extracting zip format (629Kb; 2Mb uncompressed)

  (Download the file and run it—e.g., in Windows, double-click on the file name—to get the 24 files comprising the Food Code; contents.wpd is the table of contents.)

  Note: These files were formatted using an HP LaserJet 4 printer. In order to reproduce the document as originally formatted, use of an HP LaserJet 4 printer is suggested when viewing or printing the document.

- Printed copies and computer disks from the National Technical Information Service, 5285 Port Royal Road, Springfield, VA 22161; Phone 703-605-6000 or 1-800-553-NTIS (6847)

  Spiral bound order number: PB99-115925

  Docutek order number: PB-99-115917

  Electronic Edition on CD-ROM (also includes the Adobe Reader, Draft HACCP Guide, and Plan Review Manual) (order number not yet available)

  Electronic Edition on disks (order number not yet available)

Index

Index

Page numbers followed by 'n' indicate a footnote. Page numbers in *italics* indicate a table or illustration

A

abdomen, defined 279
abdominal migraine *see* cyclic vomiting syndrome (CVS)
absorption, defined 279
Acanthamoeba 151–53
acanthamoebic keratitis 151
acanthamoebic uveitis 151
acetylandromedol 191
activated charcoal, defined 279
acute, defined 279
Aeromonas hydrophila 83
Aging, Administration on, patient drug information 268
Agricultural Science and Technology, Council for 197
Agriculture, US Department of
    egg safety 48
        mandatory testing 92
    Food and Drug Safety 265
    Foodborne Diseases Active Surveillance Network (FoodNet) 269
    Foodborne Illness Education Information Center 199

Agriculture, US Department of, continued
    frozen foods 219
        cooking 223
        grilling safety 229
        ground meat
            cooking 133, 239
            Hudson recall 132
    Meat and Poultry Hotline 31, 37, 53, 199, 217, 225, 230, 252, 303
    meat color 33
    pesticides in foods 62, 65
    public health hazards 14
    PulseNet 274, 275
    safe food preparation practices 266
AHCPR *see* Health Care Policy and Research Center, Agency for (AHCPR)
Alar (daminozide) 63
Alcohol, Tobacco, and Firearms, Bureau of
    contact information 300
    role 300
aldicarb 63, 64
alfalfa sprouts 9
    Salmonella Stanley 14
alimentary canal *see* digestive system; gastrointestinal tract

311

allergies
   defined 279
   foodborne illness symptoms 85
amanitin 175, 177, 180–81
amatoxins 176–77
amebiasis, defined 279
American Journal of Public Health 258
amnesic shellfish poisoning (ASP) 87,
   163–66
amoebas 151–53
andromedotoxin 191
Animal Health Association, US,
   guidelines for egg producers 49
animals
   Campylobacter jejuni 95
   diseases 5–6
   Salmonella 89
anisakiasis 147–50
anisakid nematodes 147
Anisakis simplex (herring worm) 147
Annals of Internal Medicine 131–32
antacids 288
   defined 280
   listeriosis 100
antibacterial sanitizers 24
antibiotics, *Campylobacter jejuni* 97
anticholinergics, defined 280
antidiarrheals, defined 280
antiemetics, defined 280
antimicrobials, Salmonellae resistance 6, 13
antispasmodics, defined 280
apple cider 7, 9
   Cryptosporidium 145
   Escherichia coli 132
   unpasteurized 55, 57
Arizona, University of (Tucson),
   kitchen pathogens 209
arthritis
   Campylobacter jejuni 97
   Salmonella 91
   Shigella 114
Ascaris lumbricoides 148
aseptic food processing, described 245
ASP *see* amnesic shellfish poisoning
   (ASP)
asymptomatic, defined 280
atrophic gastritis, defined 280
atropine 280

B

baby food, label dates 249
Bacillus anthracis 86, 103
Bacillus cereus 82, 83, 103–7
Bacillus lichenformis 104
Bacillus subtilis 104
Bacillus thuringiensis 103
bacon
   storage temperatures 29
   storage times 252
bacteria
   apple juice 55
   eggs 47
   freezer safety 220
   grilling safety 229
   infants 233–34
   kitchen safety 24, 201–8, 209–13
   lettuce 68
   slow cookers 215–16
bacteriocins, described 245
Bacteriological Analytical Manual
   145
   giardiasis outbreaks 142
   regulations for fresh vegetables 146
bag lunches safety 227–30, 231–32
Balmer, Marilyn 51
Banks, Art 238, 239, 240, 241
barium enema x-ray, described 288
   see also lower GI series
barium meal, described 291
   see also upper GI series
Batt, Carl A. 211, 213
beans, food poisoning 187–89
Beard, Charles 51
beef jerky, salmonellosis outbreaks 92
benomyl-thiabendazole 63
Benson, Charles E. 213
Bentyl (dicyclomine) 280
Berman, Adam 57
Berman, Amanda 55, 58
Berry, Bessie 217, 231, 232
Beuchat, Larry 68
biotechnology, egg safety 51
bismuth subsalicylate, defined 280,
   288
blanching, described 220–21
bleach solution, described 260

bloating, defined 280
borborygmi, defined 280
Botkins disease *see* hepatitis A
bottled water 73
  traveler's diarrhea 76
bowel, defined 280
bowel movement, defined 280
brevetoxins 163
bright light food processing 244
Broome, Claire 275
Brucella abortus 86
Brucella melitensis 86
Brucella suis 86
Buchanan, Robert 198, 203, 206
bulking agents, defined 281
Bunning, Kelly 204

C

C. perfringens see *Clostridium*
  perfringens
Campylobacter 3
  FoodNet data 270
  poultry safety measures 16–17
  reporting requirements 266
Campylobacter fetus ssp. fetus 4, 95
Campylobacter jejuni 4, 5, 16, 95–98
  see also gastroenteritis
  foodborne illness symptoms 83, 86
Campylobacter pylori, defined 281
  see also *Helicobacter pylori*
candidiasis, defined 281
canned foods
  freezer safety 219, 225
  juices 56, 59
  label dates 249–50
  regulation 14
  safety issues 23
  storage times 252
cantaloupe 8, 9
Carafate (sucralfate) 288
casseroles, storage temperatures 28
catarrhal jaundice *see* hepatitis A
cathartics *see* laxatives
cattle
  see also meat
  Campylobacter jejuni 96, 98
  Esherichia coli 5–7, 16–17

CDC *see* Centers for Disease Control
  and Prevention (CDC)
Centers for Disease Control and Prevention (CDC)
  amoebic infections 152
  bacillus outbreaks 105
  contact information 17, 296
  cryptosporidium information 146
  Food and Drug Safety 265
  foodborne diseases network 269,
    270–72
  foodborne illness database 275
  foodborne illness outbreaks 8–9,
    274
  food poisoning 39
  food safety resources 273
  gastroenteritis outbreaks 123
  Hudson frozen ground beef recall 132
  juice safety 55
  listeria incidence data 100–102
  preventing E. coli infections 133
  proper handwashing 259–60
  public health hazards 14
  role 296
  salmonella outbreaks 92
  salmonella threat 53
  sanitation in foreign countries 76
  surveillance system 11–12
cheese
  Bacillus cereus 104
  enteroinvasive *Escherichia coli* 136
  enterotoxigenic *Escherichia coli* 122
  infants 233–34
  Listeria monocytogenes 100–102
  scombrotoxin 167–68
  traveler's diarrhea 76–77
chicken *see* poultry
child care centers, food safety 253–62
children
  Campylobacter jejuni 97
  enteroinvasive *Escherichia coli* 136
  Giardia lamblia 141
  hand washing 260
  juice consumption 57
  kitchen safety 209
  mushroom poisoning 184
  pesticides 61
  Plesiaomonas shigelloides 111
  rotaviruses 160–61

chlorinated hydrocarbons 84
cholesterol
  defined 281
  eggs 50
chronic, defined 281
ciguatera toxin 43, 84
cimetidine 100
cisapride 289
City and County Health Officials, National Association of 294
Cliver, Dean O. 211, 212
Clostridium botulinum 84
Clostridium difficile, defined 281
Clostridium perfringens (C. perfringens) 83, 104, 105
cod worm 147
cold storage chart 28–29
colic, defined 281
coliforms 68
  see also bacteria
colitis
  defined 281
  pseudomembranous, defined 289
colon
  sigmoid, defined 290
  transverse, defined 290
commercial food products 10
  child care facilities 255
composted manure 8
constipation, defined 281–82
consumer education
  egg safety 47
  Escherichia coli 133
  Listeria monocytogenes 102
  seafood safety 40
Consumer Product Safety Commission, Poison Prevention Packaging Act enforcer 294
consumer trends, food processing 243–46
Contracaecum spp. 147
convenience foods
  home-based foodborne illness 198
  safety regulations 238–39
cooking safety 24–26, 240
  eggs 50
  frozen foods 223
  temperatures 30

Cooperative State Research, Education and Extension Service
  contact information 298
  role 298
coprine 175, 180
corned beef
  storage temperatures 29
  storage times 252
Corynebacterium diphtheriae 82
county extension programs 14
Coxiella burnetii 86
Crosby, Betsy 50, 51
Cryptosporidia 285
  see also parasites
  defined 282
cryptosporidiosis 71
cryptosporidium 71–74
Cryptosporidium parvum 4, 71–73, 143–46
Customs Service, US
  contact information 301
  role 300
cutting board safety 202, 204, 211–13, 254
CVS *see* cyclic vomiting syndrome (CVS)
cyclic vomiting syndrome (CVS) 282
Cyclospora cayetanensis 4, 5
  surveillance 13
cyclosporiasis 8
Cytotec (mosoprostol) 288

D

dairy products
  Salmonella 90
  Shigella 114
daminozide 63, 64
Davis, Shellee 56
day care centers
  Cryptosporidium 144, 145
  food safety 253–62
  Giardia lamblia 141
DDE 64
DDT 64
deer meat 7
defecation, defined 282
Defense, Department of, *Food Code* guidelines 238

dehydration, defined 282
delicatessen foods
  safety concerns 234
  storage temperatures 28
  storage times 252
desserts, *Salmonella* 90
DHHS Department of (DHHS),
  Health and Human Services
diarrhea
  child care centers 258–59
  defined 282
  FoodNet data 271–72
  infectious, defined 287
  traveler's, defined 290
diarrheic shellfish poisoning (DSP)
  87, 163–66
dicyclomine 280
dieldrin 64
Dietary Guidelines for Americans 50
dietitians 37
Di-Gel 280
digestants, defined 282
digestion, defined 282
digestive system, defined 282–83
  see also gastrointestinal tract
dimethyl dicarbonate 245
dinophysis toxins 87, 163
dishwashing safety 205–6, 209–13
disinfectants 260
Dispensing Information (US Pharmacopoeia) 267
distention, defined 283
disulfriram-like toxins, mushroom
  poisons 176, 180
domoic acid 87, 163
Donnatal (atropine) 280
Drug Evaluation and Research, Center for 153
Drug Evaluations (AMA) 267
DSP *see* diarrheic shellfish poisoning
  (DSP)
duodenitis, defined 283
dysentery 113, 135–36
dyspepsia *see* indigestion
dysphagia, defined 283

E

E. coli see *Escherichia coli*
education, food safety 4
EEC group *see* enteroinvasive *Escherichia coli* (EIEC)
eggs 6–7
  contamination statistics 48–49
  cookie dough 202, 205
  cooking temperatures 30
  frozen 225
  label dates 250
  pesticide regulation 62
  regulation 14, 47–49
  safety issues 47–53, 205
  Salmonella 90, 255
  Salmonella enteritidis 11, 43
  salmonellosis outbreaks 92
  shells, *Salmonella* 90
  storage temperatures 28
  storage times 251
EHEC *see* enterohemorrhagic *Escherichia coli* (EHEC)
EIA *see* enzyme immunoassay (EIA)
EIEC *see* enteroinvasive *Escherichia
coli* (EIEC)
Eilrich, Gary 66
EIP *see* Emerging Infections Program
  (EIP)
elderly
  enterotoxigenic *Escherichia coli* 122
  juice consumption 57
  Listeria monocytogenes 101
  scombroid poisoning 169
  shellfish toxins 164, 208
  Shigella 114
  thrombotic thrombocytopenic pur-
    pura 131
electrophoresis
  polyacrylamid gel 160
  pulsed-field gel 12, 273
Elkins, Edgar 66
Emerging Infections Program (EIP)
  269
Emerging Infectious Diseases (April-
  June 1995) 133
encopresis, defined 283
endoscopy, defined 283

enema, defined 283
Enriquez, Carlos 209, 210, 211
Entamoeba histolytica 285
  see also parasites
  foodborne illness symptoms 83
enteritis 96, 110
Enterobacteriacae
  foodborne illness symptoms 83
enterohemorrhagic *Escherichia coli*
  (EHEC) 129
enteroinvasive *Escherichia coli*
  (EIEC) 135–37
enteropathogenic *Escherichia coli*
  (EPEC) 125–27
enterotoxigenic *Escherichia coli*
  (ETEC) 121–23
Environmental Health Association,
  National, day-care problems 261
Environmental Protection Agency 293
  contact information 299
  Environmental Radiation Ambient
    Monitoring Systems 64
  pesticides in foods 61–62, 63, 64
  public health hazards 14
  role 299
enzyme immunoassay (EIA) 73, 160
enzymes, freezer safety 220–21
eosinophilic gastroenteritis, defined 283
EPA Journal, pesticides in foods 66
EPEC see enteropathogenic *Escherichia coli* (EPEC)
epidemic hepatitis see hepatitis A
epidemic jaundice see hepatitis A
epidemics, surveillance 14
epidemiologists, foodborne outbreak
  investigations 15
Escherichia coli (E. coli) 285
  see also bacteria
  bovine feces 8
  defined 283
  enteroinvasive 135–37
  enteropathogenic 125–27
  enterotoxigenic 121–23
  foodborne illness symptoms 83
  O157:H7 3, 4, 12–13, 129–33, 239
    apple juice 55
    FoodNet data 270, 272
    PulseNet data 274–75
    West coast outbreak 15

Escherichia coli (E. coli), continued
  outbreaks 131–32, 209
  reporting requirements 266
esophogeal spasms, defined 283
ETEC see enterotoxigenic *Escherichia
  coli* (ETEC)
ethylenethiourea (ETU) 63
ETU see ethylenethiourea (ETU)
eye diseases, amoebas 151–52

F

Farrar, Jeff 69
FDA see Food and Drug Administration (FDA)
FDA Consumer
  "A Fresh Look at Food Preserva-
    tives" 239
  "Irradiation: A Safe Measure for
    Safer Food" 51
  Safe Egg Handling 93
  "The Fright of the Iguana" 53
*FDA Desk Guide for Adverse Event
  and Product Problem Reporting* 267
fecal occult blood test (FOBT), defined 284
feces
  see also stool
  Anisakis simplex 148
  bovine 8, 72
  child care centers 257–59
  enterotoxigenic *Escherichia coli* 122
  hepatitis A 156
  oyster safety 16
  rotaviruses 160
  Shigella 113
  traveler's diarrhea 75
Federal Anti-Tampering Act 294
Federal Bureau of Investigation, Federal Anti-Tampering Act enforcer
  294
Federal Register (February 16, 1990)
  92
Federal Trade Commission
  contact information 302
  role 301
fermentation, defined 284
fiber, defined 284

filtration systems, water 74
fish
  see also seafood
  Bacillus cereus 104
  Listeria monocytogenes 99, 100
  safety issues 43–45, 240
  Salmonella 90
  scombrotoxin 167–69
flagyl 141
flatulence, defined 284
flora, intesinal, defined 287
fluoroquinolones 6
FOBT *see* fecal occult blood test
  (FOBT)
food additives 237, 243–*244
Food and Drug Administration (FDA)
  293
  amoebic infections 151, 153
  bacteria on cutting boards 213
  bar soaps for hand washing 241–42
  Consumer Information Line 198
  contact information 295
  cooking ground meat 239
  egg safety 47, 49, 50
  fish and shellfish regulations 150
  fish poisoning 169
  food analysis 101–2, 115
  Food and Drug Safety 265
  Foodborne Diseases Active Surveil-
    lance Network (FoodNet) 269
  Food Code 237, 261–62, 266, 307–8
  Food Information and Seafood
    Hotline 295
  Food Information Line 52
  food safety resources 273
  giardiasis outbreaks 142
  home based foodborne illness 197
  in-shell egg pasteurization 51
  juice pasteurization 58
  juice safety 55, 57
  listeria information 234
  MedWatch program 267
  Office of Consumer Affairs 52, 198
  outbreak of E. coli in apple juice
    products 132
  pesticides in foods 61–62, 63, 64, 65
  public health hazards 14
  PulseNet 274, 275
  regulations for fresh vegetables 146

Food and Drug Administration
  (FDA), continued
  retail food establishment inspec-
    tions 240–41
  role 294–95
  safe food preparation practices 266
  salmonella outbreaks 91
  sanitation and food protection codes
    261
  Seafood Hotline 198, 303–4
  seafood poisoning 40
  seafood safety program 41–43
  website 53
Food and Drug Officials, Association
  of 294
Foodborne Diseases Active Surveillance Network (FoodNet) 269, 270–
  72
  described 13
foodborne illnesses
  defined 284
  home-based 197–99
  juice safety statistics 55
  outbreaks
    investigations 3, 269–75
    listed 9
  prevention 16–17
    described 4
  public health challenge 3–21, 270
  reporting 31, 271–72
  statistics 269–70
Food Code
  cooking times and temperatures
    240
  egg safety 48
  food processing technology 239
  food safety routines 237–38
  obtaining 307–8
  retail food establishments inspec-
    tions 241
  retail food preparation 261–62
  seafood safety 40, 44
food color
  freezer safety 221
  safety issues 33–37
food handlers, safety issues 237–62
food labels
  juices 56–57
  use-by date 69, 247–52

Food Microbiology, bacteria in cutting boards 211

FoodNet *see* Foodborne Diseases Active Surveillance Network (FoodNet)

Food Outbreak Response Coordinating Group (FORC-G) 293–94

food poisoning 23
  see also foodborne illnesses
  statistics 39, 55
  symptoms 31, 57, 105

food preservatives 245

food product development 244–45

Food Protection, Conference for Food and Drug Safety 265
  Food Code updates 307

Food Safety and Applied Nutrition, Center for
  juice pasteurization 58
  juice safety 56
  pesticides in foods 61

Food Safety and Inspection Service (FSIS)
  Campylobacter background 98
  contact information 297, 305
  egg safety 47, 48, 49
  Food and Drug Safety 265
  Internet address 232
  listeria consumer information 102
  Meat and Poultry Hotline 37, 217, 226, 230, 232, 252
  pesticides in foods 62
  role 296–97
  safe food preparation practices 266

food safety guide 23–31

Food Safety Initiative 293

food service employees
  regulations 41, 44–45, 237–42
  traveler's diarrhea 77

food technologists 37

Food Technology, home based foodborne illness 197

FORC-G *see* Food Outbreak Response Coordinating Group (FORC-G)

fortified foods 243–44

Francisella tularensis 86

freezer burn 221
  described 34

freezer safety 27, 219–26

"A Fresh Look at Food Preservatives" 239

"The Fright of the Iguana" 53

frozen food, safety issues 23–24, 206–7, 216, 219–26
  defrosting 222–25

fruits *see* produce, fresh

FSIS *see* Food Safety and Inspection Service (FSIS)

fugu poisoning 171–74

fungicides 63

G

GAE *see* granulomatious amoebic encephalitis (GAE)

Garbus, Joel 66

gas, defined 284

gastric, defined 284

gastric juices, defined 284

gastritis, defined 284

gastroenteritis 96, 121
  see also *Campylobacter jejuni;* enterotoxigenic *Escherichia coli*
  causes 159, 257, 285
  defined 284–85
  eosinophilic, defined 283

gastroenterologists, defined 285

gastrointestinal tract
  defined 285
  foodborne illness symptoms 82–83
  mushroom poisons 176, 179

GenBank (Internet database) 93, 98, 102, 146, 162

General Accounting Office, cost of treating foodborne infections 209

genetic testing, *Escherichia coli* 12

Giardia lamblia 139–42, 285
  see *also* parasites
  foodborne illness symptoms 83

giardiasis, defined 285

GI series
  lower, defined 288
  upper, defined 291

GI tract *see* gastrointestinal tract

Gore, Al 273

Graczyk, Thaddeus K. 71

granulomatious amoebic encephalitis (GAE) 151–53
grayanotoxin 181–94
ground meat
color 35
cooking temperatures 30
Escherichia coli 130, 274
salmonellosis outbreaks 92
storage temperatures 28
storage times 252
Gulf Coast Seafood Laboratory, seafood safety program 43
Gunderson, Ellis 61
Guzewich, John 204, 205
gyromitrin 175, 177, 182

H

HACCP *see* Hazard Analysis and Critical Control Points (HACCP)
Haley, Robert 242
ham
cooking temperatures 30
storage temperatures 29
storage times 251–52
hamburgers 5–6
see also ground meat; meat
Escherichia coli 130, 131–32
food safety 202, 229, 239
hand washing 206, 231, 234
child care facilities 254, 259–60, 262
food service employees 237
regulations 41
Hazard Analysis and Critical Control Points (HACCP) 16
food safety efforts 265
home-based foodborne illness 198
juice safety 56
seafood safety 40–42, 44
HBIg *see* hepatitis B immunoglobulin (HBIg)
Health and Human Services, US Department of (DHHS) 293
Head Start Bureau 261
Health Care Financing Administration
Food and Drug Safety 265
safe food preparation practices 266

Health Care Policy and Research Center, Agency for (AHCPR)
Food and Drug Safety 265
MedWatch program 267–68
health departments, local 12
heartburn, defined 285
Helicobacter pylori
see also *Campylobacter pylori*
defined 285
treatment 291
urea breath test 291
hemolytic eremic sydrome (HUS)
Escherichia coli 130–31, 136
Shigella 114
hepatitis
causes 286, 291
defined 286
viral, defined 291
hepatitis A 155–58
child care settings 260–61
defined 286
described 155
hepatitis B
defined 286
vaccine, defined 286
hepatitis B immunoglobulin (HBIg), defined 286
hepatitis C, defined 286
hepatitis D, defined 286
hepatitis E, defined 286
hepatotoxicity, defined 286
heptatic, defined 286
herring worm 147
high performance liquid chromatography (HPLC) 166, 173
high pressure food processing 244–45
histamines 85, 167
see also scombroid poisoning
Histerothylacium 147
home economists 37
honey, food poisoning 191–94
Hoskin, George 43
hospitals
enterotoxigenic *Escherichia coli* 122
salmonellosis outbreaks 92
hot dogs
storage temperatures 28
storage times 252

HPLC *see* high performance liquid chromatography (HPLC)
Hummel, Susan 66
HUS *see* hemolytic eremic sydrome (HUS)
hydrogen breath test, defined 286
hyoscyamine 280

I

ibotenic acid 175, 178
ice cream 10, 225
  homemade 255
  Listeria monocytogenes 100
  salmonellosis outbreaks 92
IFA *see* immunofluorescent antibody assay (IFA)
IHS *see* Indian Health Service (IHS)
ileocolitis, defined 287
immune system
  amoebas 153
  drinking water safety 71
  Giardia lamblia 141
  juice contamination 57
  kidney bean lectin 187
  kitchen safety 209
  Listeria monocytogenes 101
  parasites 71
  rotaviruses 161
  salmonellosis 53
  seafood safety 207–8
  Shigella 114
immunofluorescent antibody assay (IFA) 73
Imodium (loperamide) 280
imported foods
  pesticide regulation 62
  regulation 14, 40, 57
  seafood 41–42
Indian Health Service (IHS)
  Food and Drug Safety 265
  Food Code 266
indigestion, defined 287
infant formula, label dates 249
infants
  Cryptosporidium 145
  enteropathogenic *Escherichia coli* 125, 127

infants, continued
  enterotoxigenic *Escherichia coli* 122
  food safety 233–34
  pesticides 61, 64, 65
  Plesiaomonas shigelloides 111
  rotaviruses 159, 160
  salmonellosis outbreaks 92
  Shigella 114
infectious diarrhea, defined 287
infectious hepatitis *see* hepatitis A
infectious icterus *see* hepatitis A
insulated bottles 232
InteliHealth, public drinking water 71
intestinal flora, defined 287
intestinalis 139
intestinal mucosa, defined 287
intestines
  Cryptosporidium 143–44
  Escherichia coli 129
  Eschericia coli 122
  large, defined 287
  small, defined 290
iridescent color 35
irradiation
  beef 16
  eggs 51
  food preservation 245
  meat 7
  poultry 17
"Irradiation: A Safe Measure for Safer Food" 51
isoniazid, scombroid poisoning 169

J

Jack-in-the-Box Restaurants 209
Jackson, LeeAnn 57
jaundice 155–57
  defined 287
Johns Hopkins School of Public Health
  public drinking water 71
  water treatment facilities 73
Journal of Applied Bacteriology 210
Journal of Environmental Health, diarrhea in day-care children 258–59
Journal of Food Protection, bacteria on cutting boards 211, 212

Journal of Infectious Diseases, egg safety 48
Journal of the American Medical Association, model food codes 266
Journal of the Association of Official Analytical Chemists 61, 66
juices
    see also apple cider; gastric juices; orange juice
    apple 55
    safety controls 55–59
    types, described 58–59
Justice, US Department of 301

K

Kass, Philip H. 211
keratitis, acanthamoebic 151
kidney bean lectin 187–89
kinkoti bean poisoning 187
kitchen safety 24, 201–8, 209–13
    slow cookers 215–17
Kupffer's cells, defined 287
Kurtzweil, Paula 45, 53, 199, 208

L

laboratories 12–13
Labuzza, Theodore P. 213
Lactaid 282
lactose intolerance
    Giardia lamblia 141
    hydrogen breath test 286
lamb, cooking temperatures 30
Lamblia intestinalis 139
large intestine, defined 287
lavage, defined 287
laxatives, defined 287
lectin 187–88
leftover food safety 26–27, 204, 217, 229
Leptospira 86
lettuce 9, 68–69
    see also salads
Levsin (hyoscyamine) 280
Lewis, Carol 58
Listeria monocytogenes 4, 5, 99–102

Listeria monocytogenes, continued
    foodborne illness symptoms 86
    FoodNet data 270
    infants 233–34
    statistics 100–101
    traveler's diarrhea 76
listeriosis, defined 99
liver, defined 288
liver enzyme test, defined 288
loperamide 280
lower GI series, defined 288
lunch meats
    storage temperatures 28, 227–30
    storage times 252

M

Maalox 280, 288
mahi mahi, scombrotoxin 167–69
Maine Bureau of Health, bacillus outbreaks 105–6
malabsorption syndrome 141
    defined 288
malathion 65
Maryland, University of, seafood safety program 43
mayonnaise safety 28
meat
    Bacillus cereus 104
    color 33–37
    enteropathogenic *Escherichia coli* 126
    freezer safety 221, 223
    fresh
        storage temperatures 29
        storage times 251–52
    leftovers, storage temperatures 29
    Listeria monocytogenes 100
    pesticide regulation 62
    regulation 14, 240
    safety issues 204–5
Meat and Poultry Hotline, contact information 297
meat thermometers 26
    Escherichia coli 133
    ground meat color 35
Medical Association, American
    Food and Drug Safety 265
    MedWatch reporting form 267

Medical Devices and Radiological Health, Center for, amoebic infections 153
Melon Safety Plan, salmonelosis outbreak 8
meningitis 100, 101
mercury, organic 84
metabolism, defined 288
microaerophilic organism, described 95, 96
microbes 72
food preservatives 245
kitchen safety 211
Microbiology, American Society for, foodborne infections 210
microbiology laboratories 270–71
microwave ovens
frozen foods defrosting 206
safety issues 25–26
seafood cooking 205
milk 5
Bacillus cereus 104
Campylobacter jejuni 96, 98
Escherichia coli 130
hepatitis A 156
Listeria monocytogenes 100
pesticide regulation 63, 64
regulation 14
Salmonella 90
Shigella 114
moldy food 27
mollusks 41
see also seafood
"Monitoring of Pesticide Residues..." 61
monosodium glutamate 85
Morbidity and Mortality Weekly Reports 132
bacillus outbreaks (Mar. 18, 1994) 107
diarrheal illness of E. coli (Nov. 05, 1982) 132
Escherichia coli outbreaks 132
Fugu fish poisoning (May 17, 1996) 174
gastroenteritis outbreaks 123
hepatitis A outbreaks 158
rotavirus outbreaks (Feb. 08, 1991) 162
Salmonella outbreaks 92

mosoprostol 288
MS-1 hepatitis *see* hepatitis A
mucosa, intestinal, defined 287
mucosal lining, defined 288
mucosal protective drugs, defined 288
muscarine 175, 178
muscimol 175
mushrooms
foodborne illness symptoms 82, 84
toxins 175–86
Mycobacterium tuberculosis 86
Mylanta 280, 288
myoglobin 34–35
described 33

N

Naegleria fowleri 151–53
National Institutes of Health (NIH), Food and Drug Safety 265
National Monitoring and Residues Analysis Laboratory 64
National Oceanic and Atmospheric Administration
National Seafood Inspection Program 42
role 299
seafood safety program 40, 43
National Technical Information Services, *Food Code* 308
nausea, defined 288
Navaho nation 238
nematodes 147–48
Nestlé USA, Inc., contact information 246
neurological system
foodborne illness symptoms 84, 164
mushroom poisons 176, 178–79
neurotoxic shellfish poisoning (NSP) 87, 163–66
New England Journal of Medicine 150
nicotinic acid 85
NIH *see* National Institutes of Health (NIH)
nitrite curing solutions 36
nitrites, foodborne illness symptoms 82

Nitzschia pungens 5
Norwalk-like viruses 5, 8
  oysters 39
Norwalk virus 285
  defined 288
  oysters 6–7
NSP *see* neurotoxic shellfish poisoning (NSP)
Nurses Association, American, Food
  and Drug Safety 265
nursing homes, salmonellosis outbreaks 92

O

occult bleeding, defined 288
ohmic heating, described 244
okadaic acid 87, 163
Omnibus Budget Reconciliation Act
  (1990) 267
open dating, described 247–48
orange juice 9
orellanine 175, 177
organochlorine 64
organoleptic technique 43
oxymyoglobin 35
  described 33
oysters 5–7, 39
  Plesiaomonas shigelloides 111
  safety issues 16, 205

P

PAM *see* primary amoebic meningoencephalitis (PAM)
paralytic shellfish poisoning (PSP)
  87, 163–66, 173
parasites
  Anisakis simplex 148–49
  freezer safety 220
  water-borne 71
Park, Paul K. 212
Park Service, US Interior Department, *Food Code* guidelines 238
pasta
  Bacillus cereus 104
  food safety 205, 240

Pasteurella multocida 86
pasteurization 16
  eggs 48, 51, 205
  juices 57, 58
  Streptococcus 119
pathogens 5–7
  foodborne illness 81–194
Patient Information and Education,
  National Council on 265
pectenotoxins 87, 163
Pediatrics, diarrhea in day-care children 258
penicillin, *Listeria monocytogenes* 101
pepsin, defined 289
peptic, defined 289
Pepto-Bismol 280, 288
peristalsis, defined 289
pesticides, food safety 61–66
Pharmacopoeia, US, MedWatch reporting form 267
Pharmacy, National Association of
  Boards of
  Food and Drug Safety 265
  patient drug information 267
Phenergan (promethazine) 280
Phocanema 147
phosphates, foodborne illness symptoms 84
Physicians' Desk Reference 267
phytohaemaglutinin 187–89
Pickering, L. K. 258, 259
picnic safety 227–30
Plesiomonas shigelloides 83, 109–11
Poison Prevention Packaging Act 294
polyacrylamid gel electrophoresis
  (PAGE) 160
pork 5
  cooking temperatures 30
  storage temperatures 28–29
  storage times 251–52
Postal Service, US 294
poultry 5
  Bacillus cereus 104
  Campylobacter jejuni 96, 98
  color 33–37
  cooking temperatures 30, 240
  enteropathogenic *Escherichia coli*
    126
  freezer safety 221, 223

poultry, continued
  Listeria monocytogenes 100
  pesticide regulation 62
  regulation 14
  safety issues 204–5
  Salmonella 90
  Shigella 114
  storage temperatures 29
  storage times 251–52
Preempt 51
pregnancy, *Listeria monocytogenes*
  100–102
primary amoebic meningoencephalitis (PAM) 151–53
prisons, salmonellosis outbreaks 92
produce, fresh 8, 245–46
  Cryptosporidium 145
  foodborne outbreaks 9
  hepatitis A 156
  pesticide regulation 62–63
  washing cautions 65–66, 67–69
prokinetic drugs, defined 289
promethazine 280
Propulsid (cisapride) 289
proteins
  defined 289
  eggs 49
protoplasmic poisons 176–78
pseudomembranous colitis, defined
  289
Pseudomonas aeruginosa 83, 172
Pseudoterranova decipiens (seal
  worm) 147
psilocybin 175, 178–79
PSP *see* paralytic shellfish poisoning
  (PSP)
public health
  local health departments 11–12, 270
  system, described 13–16
    see also Centers for Disease Con-
      trol and Prevention (CDC)
Public Health Laboratory Services
  (Colindale, UK), kidney bean poisoning 188
Public Health Service, US, Healthy
  People 2000 265
pufferfish poisoning 171–74
pulsed-field gel electrophoresis 12,
  273

PulseNet
  E. coli outbreak 275
  foodborne illnesses 274
  public health laboratories 273
pyloric sphincter, defined 289
pyloric stenosis, defined 289
pylorus, defined 289

Q

Quick, Robert 76, 77

R

raspberries 5, 7, 9
raw food
  enteropathogenic *Escherichia coli*
    126
  Listeria monocytogenes 100
  safety issues 24–25
  Salmonella 90
  Shigella 114
  traveler's diarrhea 76
rectum, defined 289
red kidney bean poisoning 187
reflux, defined 289
reflux esophagitis, defined 289
refrigeration
  eggs 48, 49, 52
  food storage temperature 24, 27,
    28–29, 201, 203–4, 222, 248, 253
  food storage times 251–52
Reiter's syndrome
  Salmonella 91
  Shigella 114
respiratory system
  Cryptosporidium 143
  foodborne illness symptoms 82
  shellfish toxins 164
Restaurant Association, National,
  food service workers 260–61
restaurants
  food safety regulations 238, 303
  salmonellosis outbreaks 91–92
Retail Druggists, National Association of 267
reverse transcription-polymerase
  chain reaction (RT-PCR) 160

rhodotoxin 191
rice products, *Bacillus cereus* 104–7
rotaviruses 159–62, 285
  defined 290
roundworms 147–48
Roy, Ronald 61
RT-PCR *see* reverse transcription-
  polymerase chain reaction (RT-PCR)

S

safety issues
  consumer education 4, 197–234
    egg safety 47
    Escherichia coli 133
    Listeria monocytogenes 102
    seafood safety 40
  eggs 51–52
  food color 33–37
  food guide 23–31
  food handlers 237–62
    child care settings 253–62
  governmental role 265–75
    contact information 293–305
  kitchens 201–8, 209–13
  meat color 33–37
  pesticides on foods 61–66
  seafood 39–45
salads
  see also lettuce
  see also produce, fresh
  Bacillus cereus 104
  Cryptosporidium 144
  greens, pre-washed 67–69
  hepatitis A 156
  Shigella 114
Salmonella 3, 95, 285
  see also bacteria
  defined 290
  described 53, 89–93
  eggs 47, 205, 255
  foodborne illness symptoms 83
  FoodNet data 270, 272
  kitchen safety 210
  PulseNet data 275
  Stanley 14
  surveillance 12–13
  Typhimurium definitive type 104
    (DT-104) 5, 6

Salmonella dublin 91
Salmonella enteritidus 5, 6, 7, 90–92
  described 53
  eggs 11, 48, 50, 205, 239–40
  ice cream 10–11
  statistics 266
Salmonella gallinarum 89
Salmonella paratyphi, traveler's diarrhea 76
Salmonella pullorum 89
Salmonella typhi 86, 89, 90
salmonellosis 90, 91, 211
Sanitary Food Transportation Act 294
sanitation
  child care centers 253
  enteropathogenic *Escherichia coli* 126
sausage
  storage temperatures 29
  storage times 251–52
saxitoxins 87, 163
scallions 9
school lunch safety 231–32
Science News, bacteria in cutting
  boards 211
scombroid poisoning 39, 43, 85, 167–69
scombrotoxin 167–69
Scott, Elizabeth 210
seafood
  regulation 14
  safety issues 39–45, 204–8
  Salmonella 90
  worms 147
Seafood Inspection Program, contact
  information 300
seafood retailers 40
seal worm 147
sell-by dates 247–52
septicemia 91, 100, 101
serotyping, surveillance 11–12, 269,
  275
Shalala, Donna 273, 274
shell eggs *see* eggs
shellfish
  see also fish; seafood
  Bacillus cereus 105
  foodborne illness symptoms 84, 87
  hepatitis A 156
  Listeria monocytogenes 99
  Plesiaomonas shigelloides 110

Shellfish Sanitation Conference, Interstate 42
Shellfish Sanitation Program, National 42
Shigella 95, 113–15, 135–36, 285
  see also bacteria
  foodborne illness symptoms 83
  FoodNet data 270
Shigella dysenteriae 126
Shigella sonnei 115
shigellosis
  defined 290
  enteroinvasive *Escherichia coli* 136
sigmoid colon, defined 290
sigmoidoscopy, defined 290
small intestine, defined 290
Snyder, Mary 40
Soap / Cosmetics / Chemical Specialties 242
soups, storage temperatures 28, 224
Sowards, Dan 240–41
spasms, defined 290
Spiller, Phillip 39, 40
spleen, defined 290
sponge safety 209–13
Staphylococcus aureus 82, 104, 105
State and Territorial Epidemiologists, Council of 294
State and Territorial Public Health Laboratory Directors, Association of 275, 294
State Departments of Agriculture, National Association of 294
state public health departments, surveillance 11–13, 270
stenosis 149
stews, storage temperatures 28, 224
stomach, defined 290
stool, defined 290
strawberries 9
Streptobacillus moniliformis 86
Streptococcus 117–19
Streptococcus avium 117
Streptococcus bovis 117
Streptococcus durans 117
Streptococcus faecalis 83, 117
Streptococcus faecium 83, 117
Streptococcus pyogenes 82, 117
sucralfate 288

T

Taenia saginata 83
Taenia solium 83
Tauxe, Robert V. 17
Terranova 147
tests
  cryptosporidium 73, 144
  Giardia lamblia 140
  grayanotoxin 193
  hepatitis A 156
  mushroom poisoning 184–85
  rotaviruses 160
  scombrotoxin 169
  shellfish toxins 165–66
  tetrodotoxin 173
tetradon 84
tetradon poisoning 171–74
tetrodotoxin 171–74
thiabendazole 65
thrombotic thrombocytopenic purpura (TTP) 131
Thynnascaris 147
toadstool poisoning 175
tomatoes 8, 9
Total Diet Study (FDA) 61, 64–65
toxic blooms 43
toxins
  Bacillus cereus 103
  ciguatera 43, 84
  dinophysis 87, 163
  enterotoxigenic *Escherichia coli* 122
  Escherichia coli 129
  pectenotoxin 87, 163
  saxitoxins 87, 163
  shellfish 84, 87, 163–66
  Shiga 114, 129, 131
  verotoxins 126, 129, 130, 131
  yessotoxin 87, 163
Toxoplasma gondii 86
Transportation, Department of 294
transverse colon, defined 290
traveler's diarrhea 75–77, 121
  defined 290
Trichinella spiralis 86
trimethoprim-sulfamethoxazole 101
triorthocresyl phosphate 84
triple therapy, defined 291

TTP *see* thrombotic thrombocytopenic purpura (TTP)
tuna, scombrotoxin 167–69
TV dinners
storage temperatures 28
storage times 252
typhoid fever 89, 90–91
see also *Salmonella paratyphi; Salmonella typhi*

U

United Egg Producers, egg safety 49
universal product codes (UPC) 250
UPC *see* universal product codes (UPC)
upper GI series, defined 291
urea breath test, defined 291
USDA/FDA Foodborne Illness Education Information Center
contact information 298
role 298
use-by dates 69, 247–52
uveitis, acanthamoebic 151

V

Vancouver Health Department, gastroenteritis poisoning 185
veal, cooking temperatures 30
vegetables *see* produce, fresh
venison 7
verotoxins 126, 129, 130, 131
Vibrio fluvialis 83, 172
Vibrio parahacmolyticus 5, 83
FoodNet data 270
Vibrio vulnificus 5, 43, 83
Vibro cholerae 01 5, 83

viral hepatitis, defined 291
viruses
Norwalk-like 5, 8, 39
Norwalk virus 6–7, 285, 288
rotaviruses 159–62, 285, 290
vomiting, defined 291

W

Ward, Liz 49
water
bottled 73
contaminated 8–10
Plesiaomonas shigelloides 110
Shigella 114
traveler's diarrhea 75–77
treatment 71–74
weather events, water safety 74
Welland, Diane 77
Willet, Stephanie 66
World Bank, scombroid poisoning 39
worms 147–50

Y

Yersinia enterocolitica 3, 5
foodborne illness symptoms 83
FoodNet data 270
Yess, Norma 61, 62
yessotoxin 87, 163
Young, Frank E. 262

Z

Zink, Don L. 246
zoonoses 5
Zottola, Edmund A. 211, 212

Health Reference Series
COMPLETE CATALOG

AIDS Sourcebook, 1st Edition

Basic Information about AIDS and HIV Infection, Featuring Historical and Statistical Data, Current Research, Prevention, and Other Special Topics of Interest for Persons Living with AIDS, Along with Source Listings for Further Assistance

Edited by Karen Bellenir and Peter D. Dresser. 831 pages. 1995. 0-7808-0031-1. $78.

"One strength of this book is its practical emphasis. The intended audience is the lay reader . . . useful as an educational tool for health care providers who work with AIDS patients. Recommended for public libraries as well as hospital or academic libraries that collect consumer materials." — *Bulletin of the MLA, Jan '96*

"This is the most comprehensive volume of its kind on an important medical topic. Highly recommended for all libraries." — *Reference Book Review, '96*

"Very useful reference for all libraries."
— *Choice, Oct '95*

"There is a wealth of information here that can provide much educational assistance. It is a must book for all libraries and should be on the desk of each and every congressional leader. Highly recommended."
— *AIDS Book Review Journal, Aug '95*

"Recommended for most collections."
— *Library Journal, Jul '95*

AIDS Sourcebook, 2nd Edition

Basic Consumer Health Information about Acquired Immune Deficiency Syndrome (AIDS) and Human Immunodeficiency Virus (HIV) Infection, Featuring Updated Statistical Data, Reports on Recent Research and Prevention Initiatives, and Other Special Topics of Interest for Persons Living with AIDS, Including New Antiretroviral Treatment Options, Strategies for Combating Opportunistic Infections, Information about Clinical Trials, and More; Along with a Glossary of Important Terms and Resource Listings for Further Help and Information

Edited by Karen Bellenir. 751 pages. 1999. 0-7808-0225-X. $78.

Allergies Sourcebook

Basic Information about Major Forms and Mechanisms of Common Allergic Reactions, Sensitivities, and Intolerances, Including Anaphylaxis, Asthma, Hives and Other Dermatologic Symptoms, Rhinitis, and Sinusitis, Along with Their Usual Triggers Like Animal Fur, Chemicals, Drugs, Dust, Foods, Insects, Latex, Pollen, and Poison Ivy, Oak, and Sumac; Plus Information on Prevention, Identification, and Treatment

Edited by Allan R. Cook. 611 pages. 1997. 0-7808-0036-2. $78.

Alternative Medicine Sourcebook

Basic Consumer Health Information about Alternatives to Conventional Medicine, Including Acupressure, Acupuncture, Aromatherapy, Ayurveda, Bioelectromagnetics, Environmental Medicine, Essence Therapy, Food and Nutrition Therapy, Herbal Therapy, Homeopathy, Imaging, Massage, Naturopathy, Reflexology, Relaxation and Meditation, Sound Therapy, Vitamin and Mineral Therapy, and Yoga, and More

Edited by Allan R. Cook. 720 pages. 1999. 0-7808-0200-4. $78.

Alzheimer's, Stroke & 29 Other Neurological Disorders Sourcebook, 1st Edition

Basic Information for the Layperson on 31 Diseases or Disorders Affecting the Brain and Nervous System, First Describing the Illness, Then Listing Symptoms, Diagnostic Methods, and Treatment Options, and Including Statistics on Incidences and Causes

Edited by Frank E. Bair. 579 pages. 1993. 1-55888-748-2. $78.

"Nontechnical reference book that provides reader-friendly information."
— *Family Caregiver Alliance Update, Winter '96*

"Should be included in any library's patient education section." — *American Reference Books Annual, '94*

"Written in an approachable and accessible style. Recommended for patient education and consumer health collections in health science center and public libraries." — *Academic Library Book Review, Dec '93*

"It is very handy to have information on more than thirty neurological disorders under one cover, and there is no recent source like it." — *RQ, Fall '93*

Alzheimer's Disease Sourcebook, 2nd Edition

Basic Consumer Health Information about Alzheimer's Disease, Related Disorders, and Other Dementias, Including Multi-Infarct Dementia, AIDS-Related Dementia, Alcoholic Dementia, Huntington's Disease, Delirium, and Confusional States; Along with Reports Detailing Current Research Efforts in Prevention and Treatment, Long-Term Care Issues, and Listings of Sources for Additional Help and Information

Edited by Karen Bellenir. 524 pages. 1999. 0-7808-0223-3. $78.

Arthritis Sourcebook

Basic Consumer Health Information about Specific Forms of Arthritis and Related Disorders, Including Rheumatoid Arthritis, Osteoarthritis, Gout, Polymyalgia Rheumatica, Psoriatic Arthritis, Spondyloarthropathies, Juvenile Rheumatoid Arthritis, and Juvenile Ankylosing Spondylitis; Along with Information about Medical, Surgical, and Alternative Treatment Options, and Including Strategies for Coping with Pain, Fatigue, and Stress

Edited by Allan R. Cook. 550 pages. 1998. 0-7808-0201-2. $78.

". . . accessible to the layperson."
— *Reference and Research Book News, Feb '99*

Back & Neck Disorders Sourcebook

Basic Information about Disorders and Injuries of the Spinal Cord and Vertebrae, Including Facts on Chiropractic Treatment, Surgical Interventions, Paralysis, and Rehabilitation, Along with Advice for Preventing Back Trouble

Edited by Karen Bellenir. 548 pages. 1997. 0-7808-0202-0. $78.

"The strength of this work is its basic, easy-to-read format. Recommended."
— *Reference and User Services Quarterly, Winter '97*

Blood & Circulatory Disorders Sourcebook

Basic Information about Blood and Its Components, Anemias, Leukemias, Bleeding Disorders, and Circulatory Disorders, Including Aplastic Anemia, Thalassemia, Sickle-Cell Disease, Hemochromatosis, Hemophilia, Von Willebrand Disease, and Vascular Diseases; Along with a Special Section on Blood Transfusions and Blood Supply Safety, a Glossary, and Source Listings for Further Help and Information

Edited by Karen Bellenir and Linda M. Shin. 554 pages. 1998. 0-7808-0203-9. $78.

"Recent and recommended reference source."
— *Booklist, Feb '99*

"An important reference sourcebook written in simple language for everyday, non-technical users. "
— *Reviewer's Bookwatch, Jan '99*

Brain Disorders Sourcebook

Basic Consumer Health Information about Strokes, Epilepsy, Amyotrophic Lateral Sclerosis (ALS/Lou Gehrig's Disease), Parkinson's Disease, Brain Tumors, Cerebral Palsy, Headache, Tourette Syndrome, and More; Along with Statistical Data, Treatment and

Rehabilitation Options, Coping Strategies, Reports on Current Research Initiatives, a Glossary, and Resource Listings for Additional Help and Information

Edited by Karen Bellenir. 481 pages. 1999. 0-7808-0229-2. $78.

Burns Sourcebook

Basic Consumer Health Information about Various Types of Burns and Scalds, Including Flame, Heat, Cold, Electrical, Chemical, and Sun Burns; Along with Information on Short-Term and Long-Term Treatments, Tissue Reconstruction, Plastic Surgery, Prevention Suggestions, and First Aid

Edited by Allan R. Cook. 604 pages. 1999. 0-7808-0204-7. $78.

Cancer Sourcebook, 1st Edition

Basic Information on Cancer Types, Symptoms, Diagnostic Methods, and Treatments, Including Statistics on Cancer Occurrences Worldwide and the Risks Associated with Known Carcinogens and Activities

Edited by Frank E. Bair. 932 pages. 1990. 1-55888-888-8. $78.

"Written in nontechnical language. Useful for patients, their families, medical professionals, and librarians."
— *Guide to Reference Books, '96*

"Designed with the non-medical professional in mind. Libraries and medical facilities interested in patient education should certainly consider adding the Cancer Sourcebook to their holdings. This compact collection of reliable information . . . is an invaluable tool for helping patients and patients' families and friends to take the first steps in coping with the many difficulties of cancer."
— *Medical Reference Services Quarterly, Winter '91*

"Specifically created for the nontechnical reader . . . an important resource for the general reader trying to understand the complexities of cancer."
— *American Reference Books Annual, '91*

"This publication's nontechnical nature and very comprehensive format make it useful for both the general public and undergraduate students."
— *Choice, Oct '90*

New Cancer Sourcebook, 2nd Edition

Basic Information about Major Forms and Stages of Cancer, Featuring Facts about Primary and Secondary Tumors of the Respiratory, Nervous, Lymphatic, Circulatory, Skeletal, and Gastrointestinal Systems, and Specific Organs; Statistical and Demographic Data; Treatment Options; and Strategies for Coping

Edited by Allan R. Cook. 1,313 pages. 1996. 0-7808-0041-9. $78.

"This book is an excellent resource for patients with newly diagnosed cancer and their families. The dialogue is simple, direct, and comprehensive. Highly recommended for patients and families to aid in their understanding of cancer and its treatment."
— *Booklist Health Sciences Supplement, Oct '97*

"The amount of factual and useful information is extensive. The writing is very clear, geared to general readers. Recommended for all levels."
— *Choice, Jan '97*

Cancer Sourcebook, 3rd Edition

Basic Consumer Health Information about Major Forms and Stages of Cancer, Featuring Facts about Primary and Secondary Tumors of the Respiratory, Nervous, Lymphatic, Circulatory, Skeletal, and Gastrointestinal Systems, and Specific Organs; Along with Statistical and Demographic Data, Treatment Options, Strategies for Coping, a Glossary, and a Directory of Sources for Additional Help and Information

Edited by Edward J. Prucha. 800 pages. 1999. 0-7808-0227-6. $78.

Cancer Sourcebook for Women

Basic Information about Specific Forms of Cancer That Affect Women, Featuring Facts about Breast Cancer, Cervical Cancer, Ovarian Cancer, Cancer of the Uterus and Uterine Sarcoma, Cancer of the Vagina, and Cancer of the Vulva; Statistical and Demographic Data; Treatments, Self-Help Management Suggestions, and Current Research Initiatives

Edited by Allan R. Cook and Peter D. Dresser. 524 pages. 1996. 0-7808-0076-1. $78.

". . . written in easily understandable, non-technical language. Recommended for public libraries or hospital and academic libraries that collect patient education or consumer health materials."
— *Medical Reference Services Quarterly, Spring '97*

"Would be of value in a consumer health library. . . . written with the health care consumer in mind. Medical jargon is at a minimum, and medical terms are explained in clear, understandable sentences."
— *Bulletin of the MLA, Oct '96*

"The availability under one cover of all these pertinent publications, grouped under cohesive headings, makes this certainly a most useful sourcebook."
— *Choice, Jun '96*

"Presents a comprehensive knowledge base for general readers. Men and women both benefit from the gold mine of information nestled between the two covers of this book. Recommended."
— *Academic Library Book Review, Summer '96*

"This timely book is highly recommended for consumer health and patient education collections in all libraries." — *Library Journal, Apr '96*

Cancer Sourcebook for Women, 2nd Edition

Basic Consumer Health Information about Specific Forms of Cancer That Affect Women, Including Cervical Cancer, Ovarian Cancer, Endometrial Cancer, Uterine Sarcoma, Vaginal Cancer, Vulvar Cancer, and Gestational Trophoblastic Tumor; and Featuring Statistical Information, Facts about Tests and Treatments, a Glossary of Cancer Terms, and an Extensive List of Additional Resources

Edited by Edward J. Prucha. 600 pages. 1999. 0-7808-0226-8. $78.

Cardiovascular Diseases & Disorders Sourcebook

Basic Information about Cardiovascular Diseases and Disorders, Featuring Facts about the Cardiovascular System, Demographic and Statistical Data, Descriptions of Pharmacological and Surgical Interventions, Lifestyle Modifications, and a Special Section Focusing on Heart Disorders in Children

Edited by Karen Bellenir and Peter D. Dresser. 683 pages. 1995. 0-7808-0032-X. $78.

". . . comprehensive format provides an extensive overview on this subject." — *Choice, Jun '96*

". . . an easily understood, complete, up-to-date resource. This well executed public health tool will make valuable information available to those that need it most, patients and their families. The typeface, sturdy non-reflective paper, and library binding add a feel of quality found wanting in other publications. Highly recommended for academic and general libraries. "
— *Academic Library Book Review, Summer '96*

Communication Disorders Sourcebook

Basic Information about Deafness and Hearing Loss, Speech and Language Disorders, Voice Disorders, Balance and Vestibular Disorders, and Disorders of Smell, Taste, and Touch

Edited by Linda M. Ross. 533 pages. 1996. 0-7808-0077-X. $78.

"This is skillfully edited and is a welcome resource for the layperson. It should be found in every public and medical library."
— *Booklist Health Sciences Supplement, Oct '97*

Congenital Disorders Sourcebook

Basic Information about Disorders Acquired during Gestation, Including Spina Bifida, Hydrocephalus, Cerebral Palsy, Heart Defects, Craniofacial Abnormalities, Fetal Alcohol Syndrome, and More, Along with Current Treatment Options and Statistical Data

Edited by Karen Bellenir. 607 pages. 1997. 0-7808-0205-5. $78.

"Recent and recommended reference source."
— *Booklist, Oct '97*

Consumer Issues in Health Care Sourcebook

Basic Information about Health Care Fundamentals and Related Consumer Issues, Including Exams and Screening Tests, Physician Specialties, Choosing a Doctor, Using Prescription and Over-the-Counter Medications Safely, Avoiding Health Scams, Managing Common Health Risks in the Home, Care Options for Chronically or Terminally Ill Patients, and a List of Resources for Obtaining Help and Further Information

Edited by Karen Bellenir. 618 pages. 1998. 0-7808-0221-7. $78.

"Recent and recommended reference source."
— *Booklist, Dec '98*

Contagious & Non-Contagious Infectious Diseases Sourcebook

Basic Information about Contagious Diseases like Measles, Polio, Hepatitis B, and Infectious Mononucleosis, and Non-Contagious Infectious Diseases like Tetanus and Toxic Shock Syndrome, and Diseases Occurring as Secondary Infections Such as Shingles and Reye Syndrome, Along with Vaccination, Prevention, and Treatment Information, and a Section Describing Emerging Infectious Disease Threats

Edited by Karen Bellenir and Peter D. Dresser. 566 pages. 1996. 0-7808-0075-3. $78.

Death & Dying Sourcebook

Basic Consumer Health Information for the Layperson about End-Of-Life Care and Related Ethical and Legal Issues, Including Chief Causes of Death, Autopsies, Pain Management for the Terminally Ill, Life Support Systems, Insurance, Euthanasia, Assisted Suicide, Hospice Programs, Living Wills, Funeral Planning, Counseling, Mourning, Organ Donation, and Physician Training; Along with Statistical Data, a Glossary, and Listings of Sources for Further Help and Information

Edited by Annemarie S. Muth. 630 pages. 1999. 0-7808-0230-6. $78.

Diabetes Sourcebook, 1st Edition

Basic Information about Insulin-Dependent and Noninsulin-Dependent Diabetes Mellitus, Gestational Diabetes, and Diabetic Complications, Symptoms, Treatment, and Research Results, Including Statistics on Prevalence, Morbidity, and Mortality, Along with Source Listings for Further Help and Information

Edited by Karen Bellenir and Peter D. Dresser. 827 pages. 1994. 1-55888-751-2. $78.

"...very informative and understandable for the layperson without being simplistic. It provides a comprehensive overview for laypersons who want a general understanding of the disease or who want to focus on various aspects of the disease." — *Bulletin of the MLA, Jan '96*

Diabetes Sourcebook, 2nd Edition

Basic Consumer Health Information about Type 1 Diabetes (Insulin-Dependent or Juvenile-Onset Diabetes), Type 2 (Noninsulin-Dependent or Adult-Onset Diabetes), Gestational Diabetes, and Related Disorders, Including Diabetes Prevalence Data, Management Issues, the Role of Diet and Exercise in Controlling Diabetes, Insulin and Other Diabetes Medicines, and Complications of Diabetes Such as Eye Diseases, Periodontal Disease, Amputation, and End-Stage Renal Disease; Along with Reports on Current Research Initiatives, a Glossary, and Resource Listings for Further Help and Information

Edited by Karen Bellenir. 688 pages. 1998. 0-7808-0224-1. $78.

"Recent and recommended reference source."
— *Booklist, Feb '99*

Diet & Nutrition Sourcebook, 1st Edition

Basic Information about Nutrition, Including the Dietary Guidelines for Americans, the Food Guide Pyramid, and Their Applications in Daily Diet, Nutritional Advice for Specific Age Groups, Current Nutritional Issues and Controversies, the New Food Label and How to Use It to Promote Healthy Eating, and Recent Developments in Nutritional Research

Edited by Dan R. Harris. 662 pages. 1996. 0-7808-0084-2. $78.

"Useful reference as a food and nutrition sourcebook for the general consumer."
— *Booklist Health Sciences Supplement, Oct '97*

"Recommended for public libraries and medical libraries that receive general information requests on nutrition. It is readable and will appeal to those interested in learning more about healthy dietary practices."
— *Medical Reference Services Quarterly, Fall '97*

"With dozens of questionable diet books on the market, it is so refreshing to find a reliable and factual reference book. Recommended to aspiring professionals, librarians, and others seeking and giving reliable dietary advice. An excellent compilation." — *Choice, Feb '97*

Diet & Nutrition Sourcebook, 2nd Edition

Basic Consumer Health Information about Dietary Guidelines, Recommended Daily Intake Values, Vitamins, Minerals, Fiber, Fat, Weight Control, Dietary Supplements, and Food Additives; Along with Special Sections on Nutrition Needs throughout Life and Nutrition for People with Such Specific Medical Concerns as Allergies, High Blood Cholesterol, Hypertension, Diabetes, Celiac Disease, Seizure Disorders, Phenylketonuria (PKU), Cancer, and Eating Disorders, and Including Reports on Current Nutrition Research and Source Listings for Additional Help and Information

Edited by Karen Bellenir. 650 pages. 1999. 0-7808-0228-4. $78.

Digestive Diseases & Disorders Sourcebook

Basic Consumer Health Information about Diseases and Disorders that Impact the Upper and Lower Digestive System, Including Celiac Disease, Constipation, Crohn's Disease, Cyclic Vomiting Syndrome, Diarrhea, Diverticulosis and Diverticulitis, Gallstones, Heartburn, Hemorrhoids, Hernias, Indigestion (Dyspepsia), Irritable Bowel Syndrome, Lactose Intolerance, Ulcers, and More; Along with Information about Medications and Other Treatments, Tips for Maintaining a Healthy Digestive Tract, a Glossary, and Directory of Digestive Diseases Organizations

Edited by Karen Bellenir. 300 pages. 1999. 0-7808-0327-2. $48.

Domestic Violence & Child Abuse Sourcebook

Basic Information about Spousal/Partner, Child, and Elder Physical, Emotional, and Sexual Abuse, Teen Dating Violence, and Stalking, Including Information about Hotlines, Safe Houses, Safety Plans, and Other Resources for Support and Assistance, Community Initiatives, and Reports on Current Directions in Research and Treatment; Along with a Glossary, Sources for Further Reading, and Governmental and Non-Governmental Organizations Contact Information

Edited by Helene Henderson. 600 pages. 1999. 0-7808-0235-7. $78.

Ear, Nose & Throat Disorders Sourcebook

Basic Information about Disorders of the Ears, Nose, Sinus Cavities, Pharynx, and Larynx, Including Ear Infections, Tinnitus, Vestibular Disorders, Allergic and Non-Allergic Rhinitis, Sore Throats, Tonsillitis, and Cancers That Affect the Ears, Nose, Sinuses, and Throat, Along with Reports on Current Research Initiatives, a Glossary of Related Medical Terms, and a Directory of Sources for Further Help and Information

Edited by Karen Bellenir and Linda M. Shin. 576 pages. 1998. 0-7808-0206-3. $78.

"Overall, this sourcebook is helpful for the consumer seeking information on ENT issues. It is recommended for public libraries."
— *American Reference Books Annual, '99*

"Recent and recommended reference source."
— *Booklist, Dec '98*

Endocrine & Metabolic Disorders Sourcebook

Basic Information for the Layperson about Pancreatic and Insulin-Related Disorders Such as Pancreatitis, Diabetes, and Hypoglycemia; Adrenal Gland Disorders Such as Cushing's Syndrome, Addison's Disease, and Congenital Adrenal Hyperplasia; Pituitary Gland Disorders Such as Growth Hormone Deficiency, Acromegaly, and Pituitary Tumors; Thyroid Disorders Such as Hypothyroidism, Graves' Disease, Hashimoto's Disease, and Goiter; Hyperparathyroidism; and Other Diseases and Syndromes of Hormone Imbalance or Metabolic Dysfunction, Along with Reports on Current Research Initiatives

Edited by Linda M. Shin. 574 pages. 1998. 0-7808-0207-1. $78.

"Recent and recommended reference source."
— *Booklist, Dec '98*

Environmentally Induced Disorders Sourcebook

Basic Information about Diseases and Syndromes Linked to Exposure to Pollutants and Other Substances in Outdoor and Indoor Environments Such as Lead, Asbestos, Formaldehyde, Mercury, Emissions, Noise, and More

Edited by Allan R. Cook. 620 pages. 1997. 0-7808-0083-4. $78.

"Recent and recommended reference source."
— *Booklist, Sept '98*

"This book will be a useful addition to anyone's library."
— *Choice Health Sciences Supplement, May '98*

". . . a good survey of numerous environmentally induced physical disorders . . . a useful addition to anyone's library."
— *Doody's Health Science Book Reviews, Jan '98*

". . . provide[s] introductory information from the best authorities around. Since this volume covers topics that potentially affect everyone, it will surely be one of the most frequently consulted volumes in the *Health Reference Series*." — *Rettig on Reference, Nov '97*

Ethical Issues in Medicine Sourcebook

Basic Information about Controversial Treatment Issues, Genetic Research, Reproductive Technologies, and End-of-Life Decisions, Including Topics Such as Cloning, Abortion, Fertility Management, Organ Transplantation, Health Care Rationing, Advance Directives, Living Wills, Physician-Assisted Suicide, Euthanasia, and More; Along with a Glossary and Resources for Additional Information

Edited by Helene Henderson. 600 pages. 1999. 0-7808-0237-3. $78.

Fitness & Exercise Sourcebook

Basic Information on Fitness and Exercise, Including Fitness Activities for Specific Age Groups, Exercise for People with Specific Medical Conditions, How to Begin a Fitness Program in Running, Walking, Swimming, Cycling, and Other Athletic Activities, and Recent Research in Fitness and Exercise

Edited by Dan R. Harris. 663 pages. 1996. 0-7808-0186-5. $78.

"A good resource for general readers."
— *Choice, Nov '97*

"The perennial popularity of the topic . . . make this an appealing selection for public libraries."
— *Rettig on Reference, Jun/Jul '97*

Food & Animal Borne Diseases Sourcebook

Basic Information about Diseases That Can Be Spread to Humans through the Ingestion of Contaminated Food or Water or by Contact with Infected Animals and Insects, Such as Botulism, E. Coli, Hepatitis A, Trichinosis, Lyme Disease, and Rabies, Along with Information Regarding Prevention and Treatment Methods, and a Special Section for International Travelers Describing Diseases Such as Cholera, Malaria, Travelers' Diarrhea, and Yellow Fever, and Offering Recommendations for Avoiding Illness

Edited by Karen Bellenir and Peter D. Dresser. 535 pages. 1995. 0-7808-0033-8. $78.

"Targeting general readers and providing them with a single, comprehensive source of information on selected topics, this book continues, with the excellent caliber of its predecessors, to catalog topical information on health matters of general interest. Readable and thorough, this valuable resource is highly recommended for all libraries."
— *Academic Library Book Review, Summer '96*

"A comprehensive collection of authoritative information." — *Emergency Medical Services, Oct '95*

Food Safety Sourcebook

Basic Consumer Health Information about the Safe Handling of Meat, Poultry, Seafood, Eggs, Fruit Juices, and Other Food Items, and Facts about Pesticides, Drinking Water, Food Safety Overseas, and the Onset, Duration, and Symptoms of Foodborne Illnesses, Including Types of Pathogenic Bacteria, Parasitic Protozoa, Worms, Viruses, and Natural Toxins; Along with the Role of the Consumer, the Food Handler, and the Government in Food Safety; a Glossary, and Resources for Additional Help and Information

Edited by Dawn D. Matthews. 339 pages. 1999. 0-7808-0326-4. $48.

Forensic Medicine Sourcebook

Basic Consumer Information for the Layperson about Forensic Medicine, Including Crime Scene Investigation, Evidence Collection and Analysis, Expert Testimony, Computer-Aided Criminal Identification, Digital Imaging in the Courtroom, DNA Profiling, Accident Reconstruction, Autopsies, Ballistics, Drugs and Explosives Detection, Latent Fingerprints, Product Tampering, and Questioned Document Examination; Along with Statistical Data, a Glossary of Forensics Terminology, and Listings of Sources for Further Help and Information

Edited by Annemarie S. Muth. 574 pages. 1999. 0-7808-0232-2. $78.

Gastrointestinal Diseases & Disorders Sourcebook

Basic Information about Gastroesophageal Reflux Disease (Heartburn), Ulcers, Diverticulosis, Irritable Bowel Syndrome, Crohn's Disease, Ulcerative Colitis, Diarrhea, Constipation, Lactose Intolerance, Hemorrhoids, Hepatitis, Cirrhosis, and Other Digestive Problems, Featuring Statistics, Descriptions of Symptoms, and Current Treatment Methods of Interest for Persons Living with Upper and Lower Gastrointestinal Maladies

Edited by Linda M. Ross. 413 pages. 1996. 0-7808-0078-8. $78.

". . . very readable form. The successful editorial work that brought this material together into a useful and understandable reference makes accessible to all readers information that can help them more effectively understand and obtain help for digestive tract problems." — *Choice, Feb '97*

Genetic Disorders Sourcebook

Basic Information about Heritable Diseases and Disorders Such as Down Syndrome, PKU, Hemophilia, Von Willebrand Disease, Gaucher Disease, Tay-Sachs Disease, and Sickle-Cell Disease, Along with Information about Genetic Screening, Gene Therapy, Home Care, and Including Source Listings for Further Help and Information on More Than 300 Disorders

Edited by Karen Bellenir. 642 pages. 1996. 0-7808-0034-6. $78.

"Provides essential medical information to both the general public and those diagnosed with a serious or fatal genetic disease or disorder." — *Choice, Jan '97*

"Geared toward the lay public. It would be well placed in all public libraries and in those hospital and medical libraries in which access to genetic references is limited." — *Doody's Health Sciences Book Review, Oct '96*

Head Trauma Sourcebook

Basic Information for the Layperson about Open-Head and Closed-Head Injuries, Treatment Advances, Recovery, and Rehabilitation, Along with Reports on Current Research Initiatives

Edited by Karen Bellenir. 414 pages. 1997. 0-7808-0208-X. $78.

Health Insurance Sourcebook

Basic Information about Managed Care Organizations, Traditional Fee-for-Service Insurance, Insurance Portability and Pre-Existing Conditions Clauses, Medicare, Medicaid, Social Security, and Military Health Care, Along with Information about Insurance Fraud

Edited by Wendy Wilcox. 530 pages. 1997. 0-7808-0222-5. $78.

"Particularly useful because it brings much of this information together in one volume."
— *Medical Reference Services Quarterly, Fall '98*

"The layout of the book is particularly helpful as it provides easy access to reference material. A most useful addition to the vast amount of information about health insurance. The use of data from U.S. government agencies is most commendable. Useful in a library or learning center for healthcare professional students."
— *Doody's Health Sciences Book Reviews, Nov '97*

Healthy Aging Sourcebook

Basic Consumer Health Information about Maintaining Health through the Aging Process, Including Advice on Nutrition, Exercise, and Sleep, Help in Making Decisions about Midlife Issues and Retirement, and Guidance Concerning Practical and Informed Choices in Health Consumerism; Along with Data Concerning the Theories of Aging, Different Experiences in Aging by Minority Groups, and Facts about Aging Now and Aging in the Future; and Featuring a Glossary, a Guide to Consumer Help, Additional Suggested Reading, and Practical Resource Directory

Edited by Jenifer Swanson. 536 pages. 1999. 0-7808-0390-6. $78.

Heart Diseases & Disorders Sourcebook, 2nd edition

Basic Consumer Health Information about Heart Attacks, Angina, Rhythm Disorders, Heart Failure, Valve Disease, Congenital Heart Disorders, and More, Including Descriptions of Surgical Procedures and Other Interventions, Medications, Cardiac Rehabilitation, Risk Identification, and Prevention Tips; Along with Statistical Data, Reports on Current Research Initiatives, a Glossary of Cardiovascular Terms, and Resource Directory

Edited by Karen Bellenir. 600 pages. 1999. 0-7808-0238-1. $78.

Immune System Disorders Sourcebook

Basic Information about Lupus, Multiple Sclerosis, Guillain-Barré Syndrome, Chronic Granulomatous Disease, and More, Along with Statistical and Demographic Data and Reports on Current Research Initiatives

Edited by Allan R. Cook. 608 pages. 1997. 0-7808-0209-8. $78.

Infant & Toddler Health Sourcebook

Basic Consumer Health Information about the Physical and Mental Development of Newborns, Infants, and Toddlers, Including Neonatal Concerns, Nutritional Recommendations, Immunization Schedules, Common Pediatric Disorders, Assessments and Milestones, Safety Tips, and Advice for Parents and Other Caregivers; Along with a Glossary of Terms and Resource Listings for Additional Help

Edited by Jenifer Swanson. 600 pages. 1999. 0-7808-0246-2. $78.

Kidney & Urinary Tract Diseases & Disorders Sourcebook

Basic Information about Kidney Stones, Urinary Incontinence, Bladder Disease, End Stage Renal Disease, Dialysis, and More, Along with Statistical and Demographic Data and Reports on Current Research Initiatives

Edited by Linda M. Ross. 602 pages. 1997. 0-7808-0079-6. $78.

Learning Disabilities Sourcebook

Basic Information about Disorders Such as Dyslexia, Visual and Auditory Processing Deficits, Attention Deficit/Hyperactivity Disorder, and Autism, Along with Statistical and Demographic Data, Reports on Current Research Initiatives, an Explanation of the Assessment Process, and a Special Section for Adults with Learning Disabilities

Edited by Linda M. Shin. 579 pages. 1998. 0-7808-0210-1. $78.

"Readable . . . provides a solid base of information regarding successful techniques used with individuals who have learning disabilities, as well as practical suggestions for educators and family members. Clear language, concise descriptions, and pertinent information for contacting multiple resources add to the strength of this book as a useful tool." — *Choice, Feb '99*

"Recent and recommended reference source."
— *Booklist, Sept '98*

Liver Disorders Sourcebook

Basic Consumer Health Information about the Liver and How It Works, Liver Diseases, Including Cancer, Cirrhosis, Hepatitis, and Toxic Drug Related Diseases; Tips for Maintaining a Healthy Liver; Laboratory Tests, Radiology Tests, and Facts about Liver Transplantation; Along with a Section on Support Groups, a Glossary, and Resource Listings

Edited by Joyce Brennfleck Shannon. 600 pages. 1999. 0-7808-0383-3. $78.

Medical Tests Sourcebook

Basic Consumer Health Information about Medical Tests, Including Periodic Health Exams, General Screening Tests, Tests You Can Do at Home, Findings of the U.S. Preventive Services Task Force, X-ray and Radiology Tests, Electrical Tests, Tests of Blood and Other Body Fluids and Tissues, Scope Tests, Lung Tests, Genetic Tests, Pregnancy Tests, Newborn Screening Tests, Sexually Transmitted Disease Tests, and Computer Aided Diagnoses; Along with a Section on Paying for Medical Tests, a Glossary, and Resource Listings

Edited by Joyce Brennfleck Shannon. 691 pages. 1999. 0-7808-0243-8. $78.

Men's Health Concerns Sourcebook

Basic Information about Health Issues That Affect Men, Featuring Facts about the Top Causes of Death in Men, Including Heart Disease, Stroke, Cancers, Prostate Disorders, Chronic Obstructive Pulmonary Disease, Pneumonia and Influenza, Human Immunodeficiency Virus and Acquired Immune Deficiency Syndrome, Diabetes Mellitus, Stress, Suicide, Accidents and Homicides; and Facts about Common Concerns for Men, Including Impotence, Contraception, Circumcision, Sleep Disorders, Snoring, Hair Loss, Diet, Nutrition, Exercise, Kidney and Urological Disorders, and Backaches

Edited by Allan R. Cook. 738 pages. 1998. 0-7808-0212-8. $78.

"Recent and recommended reference source."
— *Booklist, Dec '98*

Mental Health Disorders Sourcebook, 1st Edition

Basic Information about Schizophrenia, Depression, Bipolar Disorder, Panic Disorder, Obsessive-Compulsive Disorder, Phobias and Other Anxiety Disorders, Paranoia and Other Personality Disorders, Eating Disorders, and Sleep Disorders, Along with Information about Treatment and Therapies

Edited by Karen Bellenir. 548 pages. 1995. 0-7808-0040-0. $78.

"This is an excellent new book . . . written in easy-to-understand language."
— *Booklist Health Science Supplement, Oct '97*

". . . useful for public and academic libraries and consumer health collections."
— *Medical Reference Services Quarterly, Spring '97*

"The great strengths of the book are its readability and its inclusion of places to find more information. Especially recommended." — *RQ, Winter '96*

". . . a good resource for a consumer health library."
— *Bulletin of the MLA, Oct '96*

"The information is data-based and couched in brief, concise language that avoids jargon. . . . a useful reference source." — *Readings, Sept '96*

"The text is well organized and adequately written for its target audience." — *Choice, Jun '96*

". . . provides information on a wide range of mental disorders, presented in nontechnical language."
— *Exceptional Child Education Resources, Spring '96*

"Recommended for public and academic libraries."
— *Reference Book Review, '96*

Mental Health Disorders Sourcebook, 2nd Edition

Basic Consumer Health Information about Anxiety Disorders, Depression and Other Mood Disorders, Eating Disorders, Personality Disorders, Schizophrenia, and More, Including Disease Descriptions, Treatment Options, and Reports on Current Research Initiatives; Along with Statistical Data, Tips for Maintaining Mental Health, a Glossary, and Directory of Sources for Additional Help and Information

Edited by Karen Bellenir. 600 pages. 1999. 0-7808-0240-3. $78.

Ophthalmic Disorders Sourcebook

Basic Information about Glaucoma, Cataracts, Macular Degeneration, Strabismus, Refractive Disorders, and More, Along with Statistical and Demographic Data and Reports on Current Research Initiatives

Edited by Linda M. Ross. 631 pages. 1996. 0-7808-0081-8. $78.

Oral Health Sourcebook

Basic Information about Diseases and Conditions Affecting Oral Health, Including Cavities, Gum Disease, Dry Mouth, Oral Cancers, Fever Blisters, Canker Sores, Oral Thrush, Bad Breath, Temporomandibular Disorders, and other Craniofacial Syndromes, Along with Statistical Data on the Oral Health of Americans, Oral Hygiene, Emergency First Aid, Information on Treatment Procedures and Methods of Replacing Lost Teeth

Edited by Allan R. Cook. 558 pages. 1997. 0-7808-0082-6. $78.

"Unique source which will fill a gap in dental sources for patients and the lay public. A valuable reference tool even in a library with thousands of books on dentistry. Comprehensive, clear, inexpensive, and easy to read and use. It fills an enormous gap in the health care literature."   — *Reference and User Services Quarterly, Summer '98*

"Recent and recommended reference source."
— *Booklist, Dec '97*

Pain Sourcebook

Basic Information about Specific Forms of Acute and Chronic Pain, Including Headaches, Back Pain, Muscular Pain, Neuralgia, Surgical Pain, and Cancer Pain, Along with Pain Relief Options Such as Analgesics, Narcotics, Nerve Blocks, Transcutaneous Nerve Stimulation, and Alternative Forms of Pain Control, Including Biofeedback, Imaging, Behavior Modification, and Relaxation Techniques

Edited by Allan R. Cook. 667 pages. 1997. 0-7808-0213-6. $78.

"The text is readable, easily understood, and well indexed. This excellent volume belongs in all patient education libraries, consumer health sections of public libraries, and many personal collections."
— *American Reference Books Annual, '99*

"A beneficial reference."
— *Booklist Health Sciences Supplement, Oct '98*

"The information is basic in terms of scholarship and is appropriate for general readers. Written in journalistic style . . . intended for non-professionals. Quite thorough in its coverage of different pain conditions and summarizes the latest clinical information regarding pain treatment."   — *Choice, Jun '98*

"Recent and recommended reference source."
— *Booklist, Mar '98*

Pediatric Cancer Sourcebook

Basic Consumer Health Information about Leukemias, Brain Tumors, Sarcomas, Lymphomas, and Other Cancers in Infants, Children, and Adolescents, Including Descriptions of Cancers, Treatments, and Coping Strategies; Along with Suggestions for Parents, Caregivers, and Concerned Relatives, a Glossary of Cancer Terms, and Resource Listings

Edited by Edward J. Prucha. 580 pages. 1999. 0-7808-0245-4. $78.

Physical & Mental Issues in Aging Sourcebook

Basic Consumer Health Information on Physical and Mental Disorders Associated with the Aging Process, Including Concerns about Cardiovascular Disease, Pulmonary Disease, Oral Health, Digestive Disorders, Musculoskeletal and Skin Disorders, Metabolic Changes, Sexual and Reproductive Issues, and Changes in Vision, Hearing, and Other Senses; Along with Data about Longevity and Causes of Death, Information on Acute and Chronic Pain, Descriptions of Mental Concerns, a Glossary of Terms, and Resource Listings for Additional Help

Edited by Jenifer Swanson. 660 pages. 1999. 0-7808-0233-0. $78.

Pregnancy & Birth Sourcebook

Basic Information about Planning for Pregnancy, Maternal Health, Fetal Growth and Development, Labor and Delivery, Postpartum and Perinatal Care, Pregnancy in Mothers with Special Concerns, and Disorders of Pregnancy, Including Genetic Counseling, Nutrition and Exercise, Obstetrical Tests, Pregnancy Discomfort, Multiple Births, Cesarean Sections, Medical Testing of Newborns, Breastfeeding, Gestational Diabetes, and Ectopic Pregnancy

Edited by Heather E. Aldred. 737 pages. 1997. 0-7808-0216-0. $78.

"A well-organized handbook. Recommended."
— *Choice, Apr '98*

"Recent and recommended reference source."
— *Booklist, Mar '98*

"Recommended for public libraries."
— *American Reference Books Annual, '98*

Public Health Sourcebook

Basic Information about Government Health Agencies, Including National Health Statistics and Trends, Healthy People 2000 Program Goals and Objectives, the Centers for Disease Control and Prevention, the Food and Drug Administration, and the National Institutes of Health, Along with Full Contact Information for Each Agency

Edited by Wendy Wilcox. 698 pages. 1998. 0-7808-0220-9. $78.

"Recent and recommended reference source."
— *Booklist, Sept '98*

"This consumer guide provides welcome assistance in navigating the maze of federal health agencies and their data on public health concerns."
— *SciTech Book News, Sept '98*

Rehabilitation Sourcebook

Basic Consumer Health Information about Rehabilitation for People Recovering from Heart Surgery, Spinal Cord Injury, Stroke, Orthopedic Impairments, Amputation, Pulmonary Impairments, Traumatic Injury, and More, Including Physical Therapy, Occupational Therapy, Speech/Language Therapy, Massage Therapy, Dance Therapy, Art Therapy, and Recreational Therapy, Along with Information on Assistive and Adaptive Devices, a Glossary, and Resources for Additional Help and Information

Edited by Dawn D. Matthews. 512 pages. 1999. 0-7808-0236-5. $78.

Respiratory Diseases & Disorders Sourcebook

Basic Information about Respiratory Diseases and Disorders, Including Asthma, Cystic Fibrosis, Pneumonia, the Common Cold, Influenza, and Others, Featuring Facts about the Respiratory System, Statistical and Demographic Data, Treatments, Self-Help Management Suggestions, and Current Research Initiatives

Edited by Allan R. Cook and Peter D. Dresser. 771 pages. 1995. 0-7808-0037-0. $78.

"Designed for the layperson and for patients and their families coping with respiratory illness. . . . an extensive array of information on diagnosis, treatment, management, and prevention of respiratory illnesses for the general reader." — *Choice, Jun '96*

"A highly recommended text for all collections. It is a comforting reminder of the power of knowledge that good books carry between their covers."
— *Academic Library Book Review, Spring '96*

"This sourcebook offers a comprehensive collection of authoritative information presented in a nontechnical, humanitarian style for patients, families, and caregivers."
— *Association of Operating Room Nurses, Sept/Oct '95*

Sexually Transmitted Diseases Sourcebook

Basic Information about Herpes, Chlamydia, Gonorrhea, Hepatitis, Nongonoccocal Urethritis, Pelvic Inflammatory Disease, Syphilis, AIDS, and More, Along with Current Data on Treatments and Preventions

Edited by Linda M. Ross. 550 pages. 1997. 0-7808-0217-9. $78.

Skin Disorders Sourcebook

Basic Information about Common Skin and Scalp Conditions Caused by Aging, Allergies, Immune Reactions, Sun Exposure, Infectious Organisms, Parasites, Cosmetics, and Skin Traumas, Including Abrasions, Cuts, and Pressure Sores, Along with Information on Prevention and Treatment

Edited by Allan R. Cook. 647 pages. 1997. 0-7808-0080-X. $78.

". . . comprehensive easily read reference book."
— *Doody's Health Sciences Book Reviews, Oct '97*

Sleep Disorders Sourcebook

Basic Consumer Health Information about Sleep and Its Disorders, Including Insomnia, Sleepwalking, Sleep Apnea, Restless Leg Syndrome, and Narcolepsy; Along with Data about Shiftwork and Its Effects, Information on the Societal Costs of Sleep Deprivation, Descriptions of Treatment Options, a Glossary of Terms, and Resource Listings for Additional Help

Edited by Jenifer Swanson. 439 pages. 1998. 0-7808-0234-9. $78.

"Recent and recommended reference source."
— *Booklist, Feb '99*

Sports Injuries Sourcebook

Basic Consumer Health Information about Common Sports Injuries, Prevention of Injury in Specific Sports, Tips for Training, and Rehabilitation from Injury; Along with Information about Special Concerns for Children, Young Girls in Athletic Training Programs, Senior Athletes, and Women Athletes, and a Directory of Resources for Further Help and Information

Edited by Heather E. Aldred. 624 pages.1999. 0-7808-0218-7. $78.

Substance Abuse Sourcebook

Basic Health-Related Information about the Abuse of Legal and Illegal Substances Such as Alcohol, Tobacco, Prescription Drugs, Marijuana, Cocaine, and Heroin; and Including Facts about Substance Abuse Prevention Strategies, Intervention Methods, Treatment and Recovery Programs, and a Section Addressing the Special Problems Related to Substance Abuse during Pregnancy

Edited by Karen Bellenir. 573 pages. 1996. 0-7808-0038-9. $78.

"A valuable addition to any health reference section. Highly recommended."
— The Book Report, Mar/Apr '97

". . . a comprehensive collection of substance abuse information that's both highly readable and compact. Families and caregivers of substance abusers will find the information enlightening and helpful, while teachers, social workers and journalists should benefit from the concise format. Recommended."
— Drug Abuse Update, Winter '96-'97

Women's Health Concerns Sourcebook

Basic Information about Health Issues That Affect Women, Featuring Facts about Menstruation and Other Gynecological Concerns, Including Endometriosis, Fibroids, Menopause, and Vaginitis; Reproductive Concerns, Including Birth Control, Infertility, and Abortion; and Facts about Additional Physical, Emotional, and Mental Health Concerns Prevalent among Women Such as Osteoporosis, Urinary Tract Disorders, Eating Disorders, and Depression, Along with Tips for Maintaining a Healthy Lifestyle

Edited by Heather Aldred. 567 pages. 1997. 0-7808-0219-5. $78.

"Handy compilation. There is an impressive range of diseases, devices, disorders, procedures, and other physical and emotional issues covered . . . well organized, illustrated, and indexed."
— Choice, Jan '98

Workplace Health & Safety Sourcebook

Basic Information about Musculoskeletal Injuries, Cumulative Trauma Disorders, Occupational Carcinogens and Other Toxic Materials, Child Labor, Workplace Violence, Histoplasmosis, Transmission of HIV and Hepatitis-B Viruses, and Occupational Hazards Associated with Various Industries, Including Mining, Confined Spaces, Agriculture, Construction, Electrical Work, and the Medical Professions, with Information on Mortality and Other Statistical Data, Preventative Measures, Reproductive Risks, Reducing Stress for Shiftworkers, Noise Hazards, Industrial Back Belts, Reducing Contamination at Home, Preventing Allergic Reactions to Rubber Latex, and More; Along with Public and Private Programs and Initiatives, a Glossary, and Sources for Additional Help and Information

Edited by Helene Henderson. 600 pages. 1999. 0-7808-0231-4. $78.

Health Reference Series Cumulative Index

A Comprehensive Index to 42 Volumes of the Health Reference Series, 1990-1998

1st ed. 1,500 pages. 0-7808-0382-5. $78.